The Vegan Athlete's Cookbook

For Beginners

How To Improve Your Muscles And Hi-Performance Quickly.

Delicious Vegan Recipes And Protein Plant-Based Included for Your Workouts

Michael Bean

Table Of Contents

INTRODUCTION 7

UNDERSTANDING VEGAN DIET 9

BENEFITS OF VEGAN FOODS FOR ATHLETICS 17

BREAKFAST 20
    Berry and Banana Smoothie 20
    Apple Pie Smoothie 21
    Chocolate Peanut Butter and Green Smoothie 22
    Spinach Flax Protein Smoothie 24
    Chocolate Protein Shake 25
    Strawberry and Coconut Smoothie 26
    Banana Protein Smoothie Bowl 28
    Green Chocolate Protein Smoothie 29
    Chocolate and Black Bean Smoothie 31
    Super Green Smoothie Bowl 32
    Chickpea Scramble Breakfast Bowl 34
    Breakfast Grain Salad 36

LUNCH RECIPES 39
    AMAZING POTATO DISH 39
    TEXTURED SWEET POTATOES AND LENTILS DELIGHT 40
    INCREDIBLY TASTY PIZZA 42
    RICH BEANS SOUP 45
    DELICIOUS BAKED BEANS 46
    INDIAN LENTILS 48
    DELICIOUS BUTTERNUT SQUASH SOUP 49
    AMAZING MUSHROOM STEW 53
    SIMPLE TOFU DISH 54
    SPECIAL JAMBALAYA 55
    DELICIOUS CHARD SOUP 57
    CHINESE TOFU AND VEGGIES 58
    WONDERFUL CORN CHOWDER 60
    BLACK EYED PEAS STEW 61

DINNER RECIPES 63
    PESTO SPAGHETTI WITH CHICKPEA BALLS 63

- CHICKPEA, QUINOA AND SPINACH STEW 66
- TOFU SOBA NOODLES 68
- BUFFALO CAULIFLOWER TACOS 71
- TOFU STEAKS WITH SALAD 74
- SPINACH RICOTTA LASAGNA 77
- LENTIL LOAF 80
- MONGOLIAN SEITAN 83

SNACKS 87

- BEANS WITH SESAME HUMMUS 87
- CHOCO WALNUTS FAT BOMBS 88
- CRISPY HONEY PECANS (SLOW COOKER) 91
- CRUNCHY FRIED PICKLES 92
- GRANOLA BARS WITH MAPLE SYRUP 93
- GREEN SOY BEANS HUMMUS 95
- HIGH PROTEIN AVOCADO GUACAMOLE 97
- HOMEMADE ENERGY NUT BARS 99
- HONEY PEANUT BUTTER 100
- MEDITERRANEAN MARINATED OLIVES 102

PASTA RECIPES 105

- MUSHROOM CREAM SAUCE PASTA 105
- PENNE WITH BLACK BEANS AND VEGETABLES 108
- TOFU PENNE PASTA 110
- SPINACH GARLIC PASTA 112
- LINGUINE WITH GUACAMOLE 113

DESSERT RECIPES 115

- BANANA-NUT BREAD BARS 115
- LEMON COCONUT CILANTRO ROLLS 116
- TAMARI ALMONDS 117
- TEMPEH TACO BITES 118
- STUFFED CHERRY TOMATOES 122
- SPICY BLACK BEAN DIP 123
- CHEEZY CASHEW–ROASTED RED PEPPER TOASTS 124
- BAKED POTATO CHIPS 125
- MUSHROOMS STUFFED WITH SPINACH AND WALNUTS 127
- SALSA FRESCA 128
- GUACAMOLE 129
- ASIAN LETTUCE ROLLS 130

CONCLUSION 132

© Copyright 2020 by Michael Bean - All rights reserved.

The following Book is reproduced below with the goal of providing information that is as accurate and reliable as possible. Regardless, purchasing this Book can be seen as consent to the fact that both the publisher and the author of this book are in no way experts on the topics discussed within and that any recommendations or suggestions that are made herein are for entertainment purposes only. Professionals should be consulted as needed prior to undertaking any of the action endorsed herein.

This declaration is deemed fair and valid by both the American Bar Association and the Committee of Publishers Association and is legally binding throughout the United States.

Furthermore, the transmission, duplication, or reproduction of any of the following work including specific information will be considered an illegal act irrespective of if it is done electronically or in print. This extends to creating a secondary or tertiary copy of the work or a recorded copy and is only allowed with the express written consent from the Publisher. All additional right reserved.

The information in the following pages is broadly considered a truthful and accurate account of facts and as such, any inattention, use, or misuse of the information in question by the reader will render any resulting actions solely under their purview. There are no scenarios in which the publisher or the original author of this work can be in any fashion deemed liable for any hardship or damages that may befall them after undertaking information described herein.

Additionally, the information in the following pages is intended only for informational purposes and should thus be thought of as universal. As befitting its nature, it is presented without assurance regarding its prolonged validity or interim quality. Trademarks that are mentioned are done without written consent and can in no way be considered an endorsement from the trademark holder.

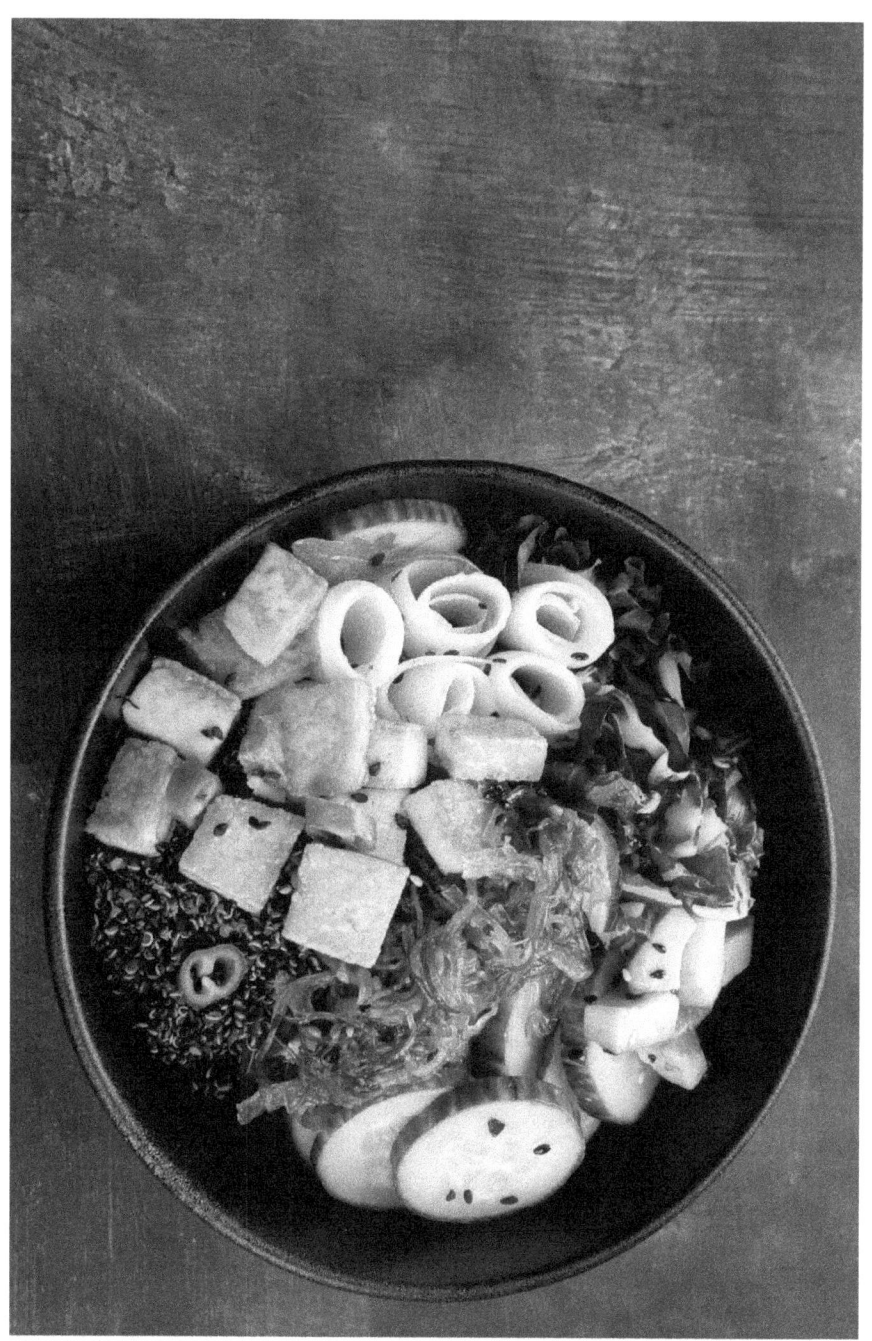

Introduction

People are doing their best to change their fast consumption lifestyle, and one way to change that is becoming vegan. Veganism is not just an ethical choice for the lives of the animals; it is also an eco-friendly choice. Our planet is dying rapidly, and it will take a lot of effort for damage control. But like they say every small step helps, so you can do your bit by turning to veganism. The meat industry or livestock farming as it is called has a huge adverse impact on the environment. It contributes to about 18% of the greenhouse gases, which is a huge number. Turning vegan can definitely help lighten that burden and accelerate our growth towards damage control.

It is not only for this reason that people switch to a vegan lifestyle. There are numerous benefits to the vegan diet, which are explained in detail in the first chapter of the book. There is a strong misconception that the vegan diet lacks substantial protein, and hence it is not ideal for athletes and bodybuilder. Well, in all honesty, it is nothing but a misconception. Athletes can switch to a vegan diet; they just need to identify healthier substitutes for the animal protein, and there are plenty of options.

Plant foods offer a wide range of advantages over animal foods. They are scientifically recommended for healthy living as they promote a person's wellbeing. By eating plant-based foods, a person is able to reduce the risk of certain illnesses and avoid problems associated with overweight/obesity.

Plant foods are advantageous in their low fat and calorie load. They are also dense in their protein content. Proteins are excellent in helping a person watch weight as they prevent the gaining of body fat. By consuming plant proteins, a person produces more weight limiting hormones. Proteins also help in weight reduction by reducing the feelings of hunger while at the same time increasing the metabolic rate of the body.

Understanding Vegan Diet

Veganism is not just another newfangled diet or passing fad. Plant-based and animal product–free diets have been around for centuries. Even the term "vegan" has been in circulation for decades. In the 1940s, several members of England's then nearly one-hundred-year-old Vegetarian Society split off to form their own organization that focused on a strictly plant-based diet that eschewed all animal-derived foods. These strict vegetarians chose the name "vegan" because, as one of the founding members of the first Vegan Society, Donald Watson, said, "veganism starts with vegetarianism and carries it through to its logical conclusion."

A vegan diet can be defined as a "total vegetarian" diet, meaning one that is entirely plant-based and omits all animal products, including meat, eggs, dairy, honey, gelatin, and other products that come from animals. Vegans eat a plant-based diet of vegetables, grains, legumes, fruits, nuts, and seeds.

Veganism, however, is much more than a diet. It is a way of life. Those who choose a vegan lifestyle not only eat plant-based foods but also choose not to purchase products made from leather, wool, silk, and down, including cosmetics and soaps that contain animal products or are tested on animals.

Why We Eat Vegan

While there are many reasons why people choose veganism—allergies, specific health concerns, and personal preference, among others—one of the main drives is a desire for a "cruelty-free" lifestyle that avoids exploiting animals and seeks to create a more humane society. Choosing to eat only plant-based foods is a decisive way to reduce animal suffering. And if your decision to become a vegan influences others to do the same, the effect is exponential.

Being vegan also helps the environment, since raising animals for food requires vital resources such as food and water, and in many cases, trees need to be razed to make room for ranches. Animal waste also contaminates the soil, air, and water. So great is the damage done to the environment by the meat industry that the Union of Concerned Scientists considers meat eating to be one of the biggest environmental hazards we face today, second only to our reliance on fossil-fueled vehicles.

Another popular reason for adopting a vegan diet is good health. A well-balanced vegan diet can be extremely healthy since it includes plenty of fruit, vegetables, whole grains, nuts, and seeds, making it rich in vitamins, antioxidants, and fiber.

Furthermore, by eating only plant-based foods, you automatically eliminate cholesterol and unhealthy saturated fats. Adhering to a well-balanced vegan diet can decrease the risk of developing many diseases, including diabetes, heart disease, stroke, and some types of cancer.

Vegans tend to be thinner and fitter than their meat- and/or dairy-eating counterparts, too. Just look at all the glamorous celebrities who have chosen this lifestyle: Ellen DeGeneres, Shania Twain, Casey Affleck, Tobey Maguire, Alicia Silverstone, Kristen Bell, Alyssa Milano, Joss Stone, Anne Hathaway, Michelle Pfeiffer, and Carrie Underwood, to name a few.

Finally, eating a plant-based diet is economical. The diet is centered on whole grains, legumes, fruits, vegetables, nuts, and seeds—all of which are generally much less expensive than meat or dairy products, especially when purchased in season.

Guidelines and Rules for Eating Vegan

A vegan diet can be a very healthy way of eating, as long as it's well balanced to ensure that you're getting the right mix of nutrients. Since veganism eliminates all animal-derived foods, it can be a bit of a challenge to meet your daily needs for certain nutrients that are primarily found in animal products, such as vitamin B12, vitamin D, calcium, iron, iodine, omega-3 fatty acids, zinc, and even protein.

Eat Your Veggies (and Fruits)

Every good diet starts with eating the recommended five or more servings of fruits and vegetables each day. This ensures that you get a wide range of vitamins, minerals, and antioxidants. These are the ingredients of a healthy diet and the nutrients that decrease your risk of diseases like heart disease, stroke, and many types of cancer. Of course, if your diet is solely plant-based, this part is a piece of cake (vegan cake, of course)!

Calcium

Calcium, which is crucial for building and maintaining strong bones and healthy muscles and nerves, is most commonly derived from animal products such as milk and other dairy products, but dark and leafy green vegetables—think kale, chard, collard greens, and broccoli—can provide sufficient quantities of calcium if you eat enough of them. You can also buy calcium-fortified juices, breads, cereals, soy milk, and other products to make sure you're getting enough. Most adults should consume 1,000 to 1,200 milligrams per day of calcium, either through food sources or as supplements.

Iodine

Iodine is another important nutrient that keeps your thyroid running smoothly. While many food sources of iodine are animal-based (dairy products, eggs, and fish), high concentrations can also be found in sea vegetables and strawberries. Iodized salt is fortified with iodine. Most adults need about 150 micrograms of iodine per day.

Iron

Iron is essential for developing red blood cells. Iron from meat is the most easily absorbed by the human body, but there are many plant-based sources of iron as well. Dried beans, iron-fortified cereals and breads, whole-grain foods, dark and leafy green vegetables, and dried fruit all contain ample amounts of iron. To maximize your absorption of the iron in these foods, combine them with rich sources of vitamin C, such as strawberries, citrus fruits, tomatoes, cabbage, and broccoli.

Omega-3 Fatty Acids

Omega-3 fatty acids help regulate metabolism and reduce the risk of cardiovascular disease. The most common dietary sources of these essential fatty acids are fish and eggs, but they can be found in canola oil or soy oil, walnuts, flaxseed, and soybeans.

Vitamin B12

Vitamin B12 is vitally important because it plays a key role in cell metabolism, the normal functioning of the brain and nervous system, and the formation of blood. It's found naturally in animal-based foods, including meat, fish, poultry, eggs, and dairy products, but many vegan-friendly foods are fortified with a synthetic form of vitamin B12, including soy milk and breakfast cereals. Supplements are also available in the form of pills, sublinguals, or injections. Aim to eat at least 3 micrograms per day in fortified foods or take a 10-microgram supplement daily.

Vitamin D

Like calcium, vitamin D is important for maintaining healthy bones. Many nondairy milks, however, are also fortified with vitamin D, as are many cereals and breads. Most adults need a minimum of 200 to 400 international units of vitamin D each day.

Zinc

Zinc plays a critical role in keeping the immune system strong as well as in cell division and the formation of proteins. Like iron, zinc from plant sources is not absorbed by the body as easily as that from animal products such as dairy. Good vegan sources of zinc include soybeans and products made with soybeans (such as tofu), whole grains, legumes, nuts, and wheat germ.

What to Eat

In the simplest terms, sticking to a vegan diet means eating only plant-based foods. So what does that mean in practice? It means you can eat cooked and raw vegetables and fruits, grains, vegetable oils, legumes (beans, peas, lentils, peanuts), nuts and nut butters, seeds and seed butters, cereals, eggless noodles and pasta, and baked goods such as breads, cookies, and cakes (so long as they are made without animal products). Here are just some of the foods available to you on a vegan diet:

Vegetables: asparagus, beets, broccoli, Brussels sprouts, cauliflower, chard, corn, cucumbers, eggplant, kale, lettuce, olives, onions, parsnips, potatoes, radishes, squash, sweet potatoes/yams, tomatoes, turnips

Fruits: apples, bananas, blackberries, blueberries, cherries, coconuts, grapes, mangos, melons, nectarines, papayas, peaches, pineapples, plums, raspberries, strawberries

Grains: amaranth, barley, farro, oats, quinoa, rice, wheat, and other grains; grain-based foods such as baked goods, breads, couscous, noodles (eggless)

Legumes: beans, lentils, peanuts and peanut butter, peas, soy products (tofu, miso, soy sauce, etc.)

Nondairy milks: almond milk, cashew milk, coconut cream, coconut milk, hemp milk, rice milk, soy milk

Nuts and nut butters: almonds, almond butter, cashews, cashew butter, hazelnuts, hazelnut butter, pecans, walnuts

Oils: avocado, canola, coconut, flaxseed, grapeseed, olive, sesame

Seeds and seed butters: chia seeds, flaxseed, pine nuts, pumpkin seeds (pepitas), sesame seeds, tahini (sesame seed paste)

Sweeteners: agave nectar, fruit, maple syrup, stevia, sugar (some sugars use animal products, so make sure you buy vegan sugar)

Vegan substitutes: coconut butter, meatless deli slices, soy- or wheat gluten–based faux meat products such as tofu hot dogs, vegan cheese made from either nuts or tapioca, vegan egg replacer, vegan margarine, vegan mayonnaise, veggie burgers

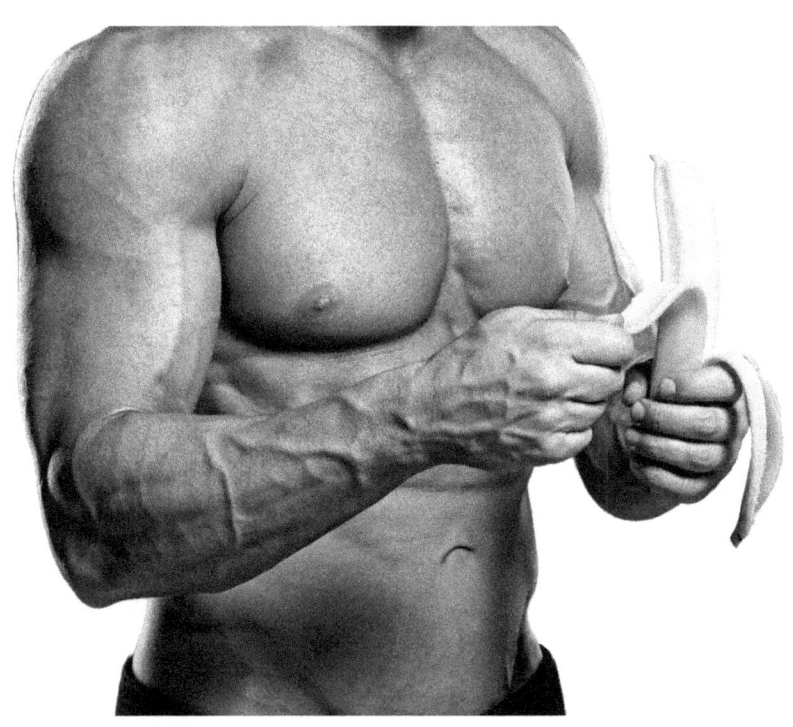

Benefits Of Vegan Foods For Athletics

Athletes nowadays are running towards veganism because they know of its benefits. Some of these benefits include:
It keeps heart healthy
Athletes need to keep the heart-healthy as well. Exercising throughout the day decreases a lot of diseases, but some linger on. A study showed that almost half of the runners and cyclists develop heart diseases and coronary plugs. Coronary plugs are caused by fat accumulation in the arteries. When athletes convert to veganism, it reduces the chances of heart disease significantly. This increased their motility and quality of life. By taking good fats in the form of avocados and seeds, the level of bad fats goes down that causes coronary plugs and heart disease.
It reduces pain intensity
When going through an intense workout, muscles develop lactic acid and go through the inflammation process, which causes a lot of pain. If an athlete converts to veganism, they experience less pain and better recovery from exercise. This is due to the anti-inflammatory effects of plant-based foods. Numerous studies have been done to show the anti-inflammatory effects of vegan dieting. It has also been proven that meat consumption and high cholesterol level contributes to the inflammatory reaction. For an athlete, a quick recovery from an exercise can mean a lot of progress.
It improves the circulation of oxygen

During exercise, the blood must provide adequate energy and oxygen to all parts of the body, including muscles. When consuming red meat and high cholesterol in the form of animal fat, blood cholesterol, and the fat level goes high. This causes the blood to thicken and becomes hard to pump. This causes much strain on the heart as well. By converting to veganism, the person can provide adequate oxygen circulation around the body by lowering cholesterol and fat levels.

It makes arterial functions work better

When consuming meat and high cholesterol meals, it was seen that that arterial function was impaired for several hours even after one meal. When consuming plant-based foods, the function of arteries becomes better. Blood becomes easy to flow due to arteries being more flexible and the diameter wider. Arterial flexibility is linked with plant-based foods, so eating more plants will make your arteries more flexible and blood flow easier.

It provides the body with antioxidants

One of the most promising results in dieting in athletes is their ability to recover quickly and feel less fatigued. This is possible due to plant-based foods replacing the cholesterol and fatty animal-based ones. During exercise, the body releases many free radicals, which are cause for concern. They move freely and damage the surrounding structures. Antioxidants neutralize these free radicals and prevent them from doing any damage.

It increases the endurance of athletes

When consuming animal-based food, body fat level tends to rise. When a person converts to veganism, the body fat levels start to sink. This leads to a higher oxygen-carrying capacity. In a study, it was shown that people following a vegan diet have a higher VO2 level, which means they can use oxygen during exercise and increase their endurance.

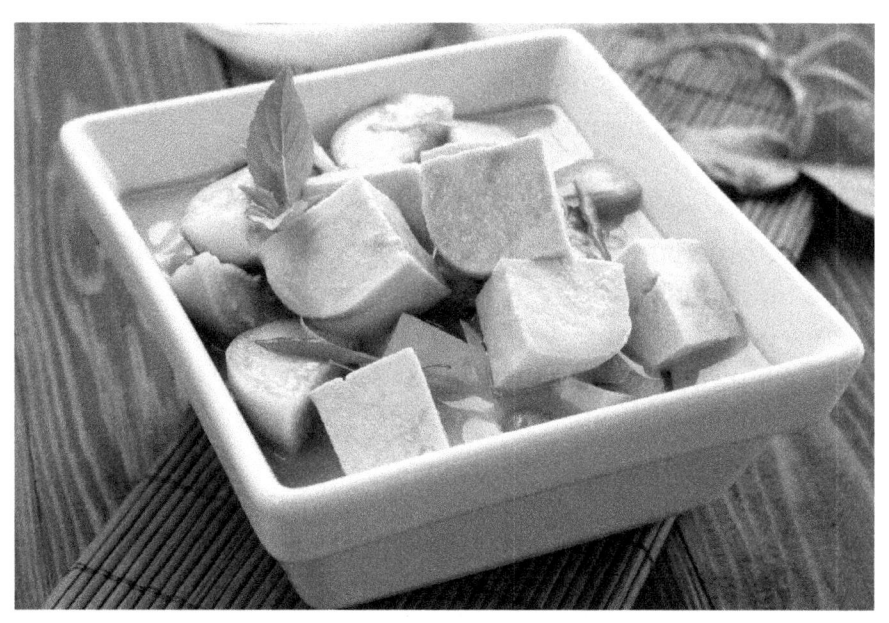

Breakfast

Berry and Banana Smoothie

Serving: 4
Nutrition:
200.1 Cal; 2.7 g Fat; 0.4 g Saturated Fat; 35.6 g Carbohydrates; 6.3 g Fiber; 22 g Sugars; 13 g Protein;
Preparation time: 5 minutes
Cooking time: 0 minutes
Ingredients:
½ cup flaxseeds
5 cups frozen berry
4 medium bananas
2 cups baby spinach
1/2-inch piece of ginger, peeled
4 tablespoons walnuts
5 cups of water
Directions:
Add all the ingredients in the order into a food processor and blender and then pulse for 1 to 2 minutes until blended. Distribute the smoothie among glasses and then serve.

Apple Pie Smoothie

Serving: 4
Nutrition:
211.7 Cal; 6.2 g Fat; 1.23 g Saturated Fat; 23.6 g Carbohydrates; 5.3 g Fiber; 8.3 g Sugars; 15.7 g Protein;
Preparation time: 5 minutes
Cooking time: 0 minutes
Ingredients:
2.1 ounces rolled oats
4 apples, cored, diced
4 tablespoons chia seeds
1 teaspoon stevia
4 scoops of vanilla protein powder, vegan
1 teaspoon ground nutmeg
1 teaspoon ground cinnamon
17 ounces coconut yogurt
4 cups almond milk, unsweetened
Directions:
Add all the ingredients in the order into a food processor and blender and then pulse for 1 to 2 minutes until blended. Distribute the smoothie among glasses and then serve.

Chocolate Peanut Butter and Green Smoothie

Serving: 2
Nutrition:
298 Cal; 7.6 g Fat; 1 g Saturated Fat; 56 g Carbohydrates; 10 g Fiber; 30 g Sugars; 9 g Protein;
Preparation time: 5 minutes
Cooking time: 0 minutes
Ingredients:
3 Medjool dates pitted
2 cups frozen spinach
2 tablespoons oats, old-fashioned
1 frozen banana
2 cups frozen kale
1 tablespoon cocoa powder, unsweetened
1 tablespoon peanut butter
1 ½ cups vanilla almond milk, unsweetened
Directions:
Add all the ingredients in the order into a food processor and blender and then pulse for 1 to 2 minutes until blended. Distribute the smoothie among glasses and then serve.

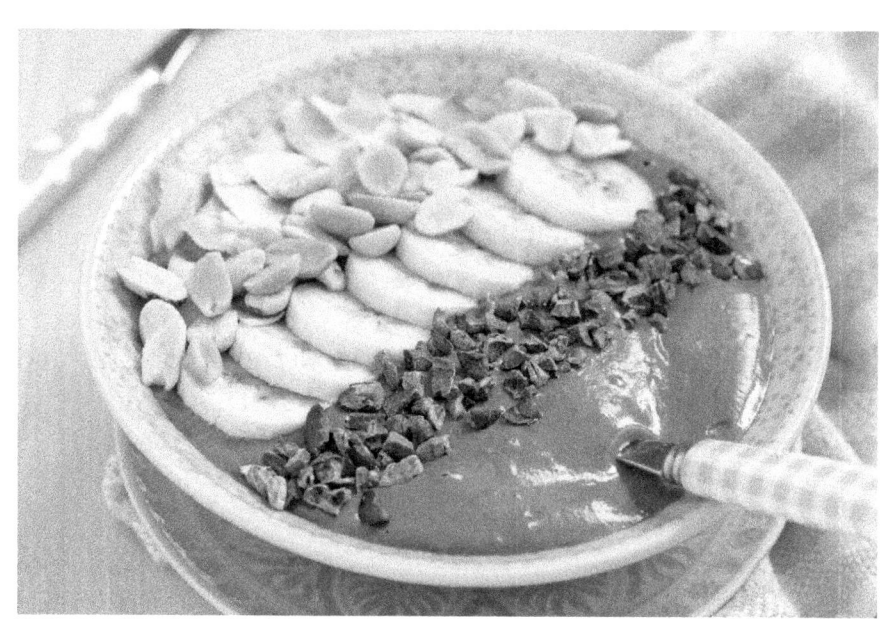

Spinach Flax Protein Smoothie

Serving: 2
Nutrition:
257.5 Cal; 6 g Fat; 0.1 g Saturated Fat; 36.7 g Carbohydrates; 8.1 g Fiber; 17.2 g Sugars; 14.2 g Protein;
Preparation time: 5 minutes
Cooking time: 0 minutes
Ingredients:
2 cups baby spinach
½ cup frozen mango chunks
2 tablespoons chia seeds
½ cup frozen pineapple
2 tablespoons flax meal
1 banana, peeled
2 scoops of vanilla protein powder
2 cups almond milk, unsweetened
Directions:
Add all the ingredients in the order into a food processor and blender and then pulse for 1 to 2 minutes until blended. Distribute the smoothie among glasses and then serve.

Chocolate Protein Shake

Serving: 2
Nutrition:
396 Cal; 11 g Fat; 1 g Saturated Fat; 68 g Carbohydrates; 15 g Fiber; 28 g Sugars; 14 g Protein;
Preparation time: 5 minutes
Cooking time: 0 minutes
Ingredients:
8 frozen bananas, sliced
4 tablespoons chia seeds
1 cup peanut flour
4 cups chocolate almond milk, unsweetened
Directions:
Add all the ingredients in the order into a food processor and blender and then pulse for 1 to 2 minutes until blended. Distribute the smoothie among glasses and then serve.

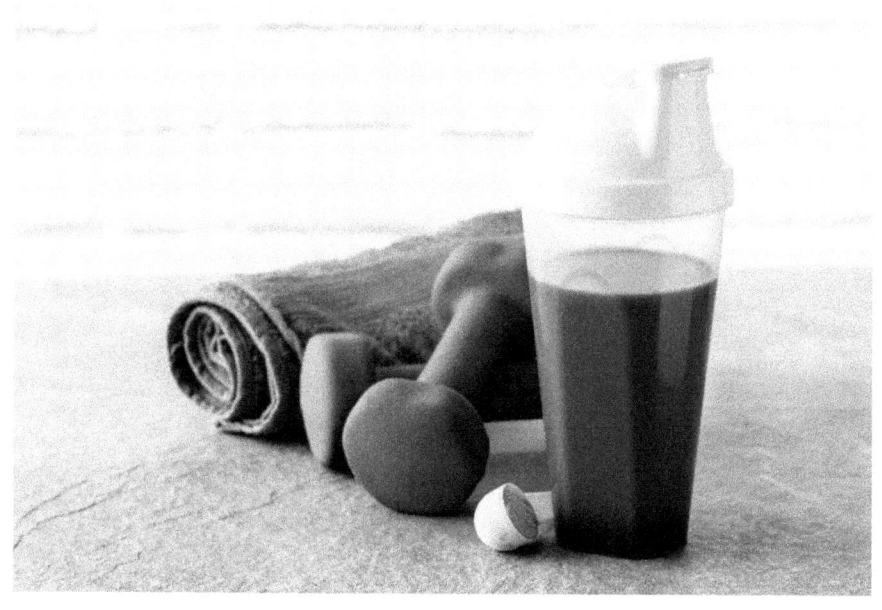

Strawberry and Coconut Smoothie

Serving: 2
Nutrition:
270 Cal; 7 g Fat; 2 g Saturated Fat; 31 g Carbohydrates; 8 g Fiber; 22 g Sugars; 21 g Protein;
Preparation time: 5 minutes
Cooking time: 0 minutes
Ingredients:
2 cups frozen strawberries
2 teaspoons ground flax seed
1/2 cup vanilla protein powder
4 teaspoons honey
2 teaspoons vanilla extract, unsweetened
2 cups coconut milk, unsweetened
Directions:
Add all the ingredients in the order into a food processor and blender and then pulse for 1 to 2 minutes until blended. Distribute the smoothie among glasses and then serve.

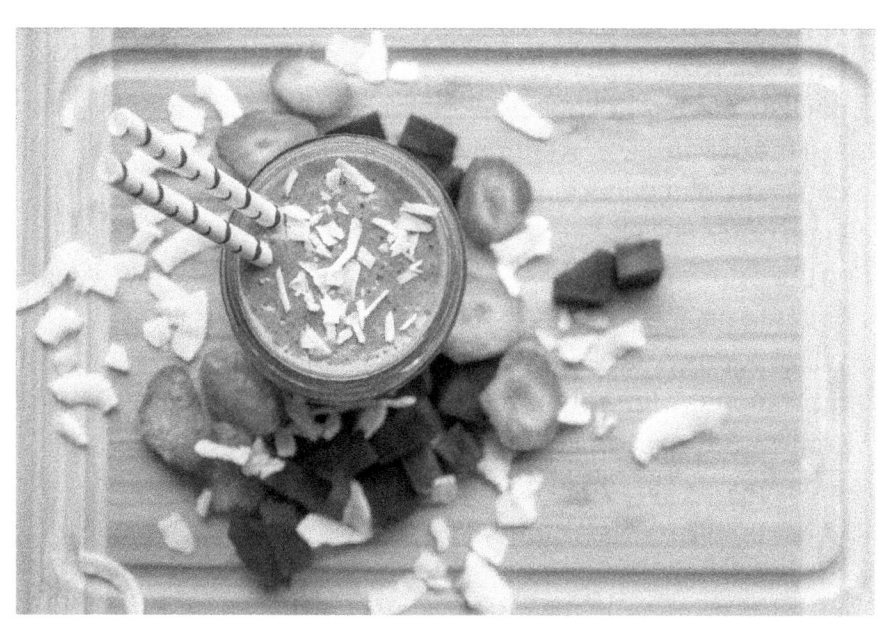

Banana Protein Smoothie Bowl

Serving: 2
Nutrition:
272 Cal; 4 g Fat; 1 g Saturated Fat; 45 g Carbohydrates; 7.2 g Fiber; 26.6 g Sugars; 20 g Protein;
Preparation time: 5 minutes
Cooking time: 0 minutes
Ingredients:
For the Bowl:
2 large frozen bananas
2 cups spinach
2 packets of instant coffee
2 scoops of vanilla protein powder
2 cups chocolate almond milk
½ cup of ice cubes
For the Topping:
1 banana, peeled, sliced
2 tablespoons chia seeds
2 tablespoons almond butter
½ cup sliced strawberries
2 tablespoons shredded coconut, unsweetened
2 tablespoons toasted almonds
Directions:
Add all the ingredients for the bowl in the order into a food processor and blender and then pulse for 1 to 2 minutes until blended.
Distribute the smoothie between the bowls, then top evenly with banana slices, chia seeds, almond butter, strawberries, coconut, and almonds and then serve.

Green Chocolate Protein Smoothie

Serving: 4
Nutrition:
290 Cal; 3 g Fat; 1 g Saturated Fat; 37 g Carbohydrates; 9 g Fiber; 23 g Sugars; 34 g Protein;
Preparation time: 5 minutes
Cooking time: 0 minutes
Ingredients:
3 large Medjool dates, pitted
1 large frozen banana
1 cup of frozen organic kale
2 tablespoons chopped avocado
2 tablespoons cocoa powder, unsweetened
2 tablespoons hemp seeds, hulled
1/8 teaspoon cinnamon
1 1/2 cups almond milk, unsweetened
½ cup of ice cubes
Directions:
Add all the ingredients in the order into a food processor and blender and then pulse for 1 to 2 minutes until blended. Distribute the smoothie among glasses and then serve.

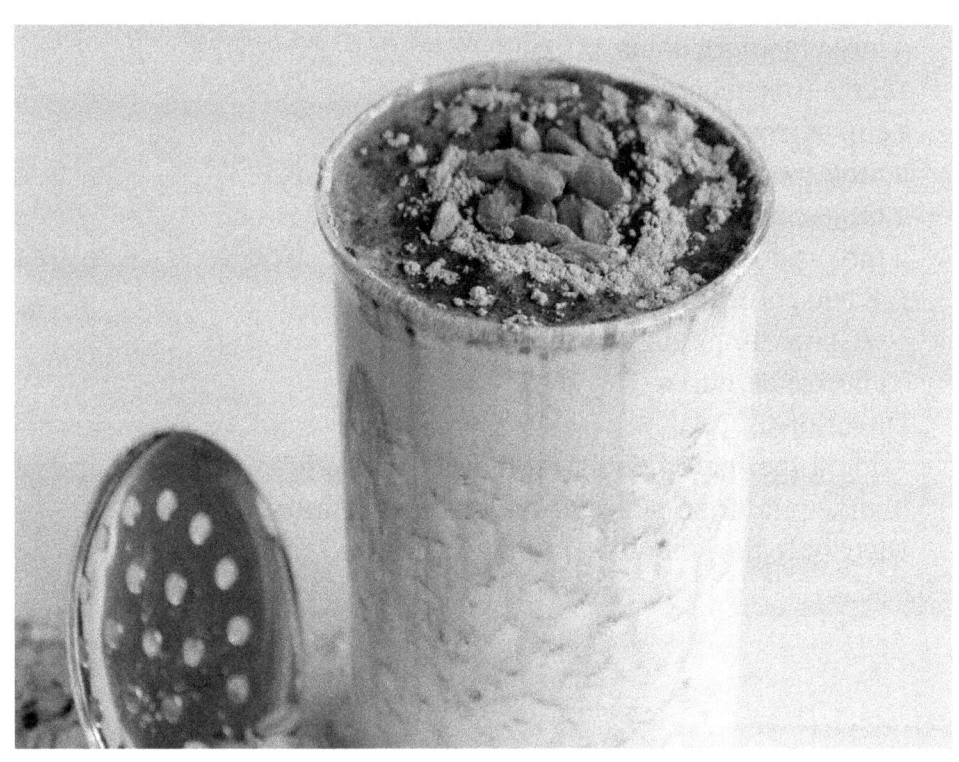

Chocolate and Black Bean Smoothie

Serving: 4
Nutrition:
226 Cal; 5.5 g Fat; 0.5 g Saturated Fat; 38.5 g Carbohydrates; 9 g Fiber; 16 g Sugars; 9.5 g Protein;
Preparation time: 5 minutes
Cooking time: 0 minutes
Ingredients:
1 cup cooked black beans
2 frozen banana
4 Medjool dates pitted
2 cup frozen cauliflower
2 teaspoons ground cinnamon
2 tablespoons hemp seeds
2 tablespoons cocoa powder, unsweetened
2 cup almond milk, unsweetened
Directions:
Add all the ingredients in the order into a food processor and blender and then pulse for 1 to 2 minutes until blended. Distribute the smoothie among glasses and then serve.

Super Green Smoothie Bowl

Serving: 2
Nutrition:
310 Cal; 15.6 g Fat; 1.9 g Saturated Fat; 41.5 g Carbohydrates; 9.5 g Fiber; 19 g Sugars; 7.9 g Protein;
Preparation time: 5 minutes
Cooking time: 0 minutes
Ingredients:
For the Bowl:
1 cup of frozen mixed berries
1/4 of a medium avocado
1 tablespoon flaxseed meal
2 frozen bananas
2 cups spinach
4 tablespoons peanut butter
1 cup kale
2 cups almond milk, unsweetened
For the Topping:
2 tablespoons hemp seeds
2 tablespoons sunflower seeds
2 tablespoons shredded coconut, unsweetened
¼ cup sliced berries
Directions:
Add all the ingredients for the bowl in the order into a food processor and blender and then pulse for 1 to 2 minutes until blended.
Distribute the smoothie between the bowls, then top evenly with hemp seeds, sunflower seeds, coconut, and berries and then serve.

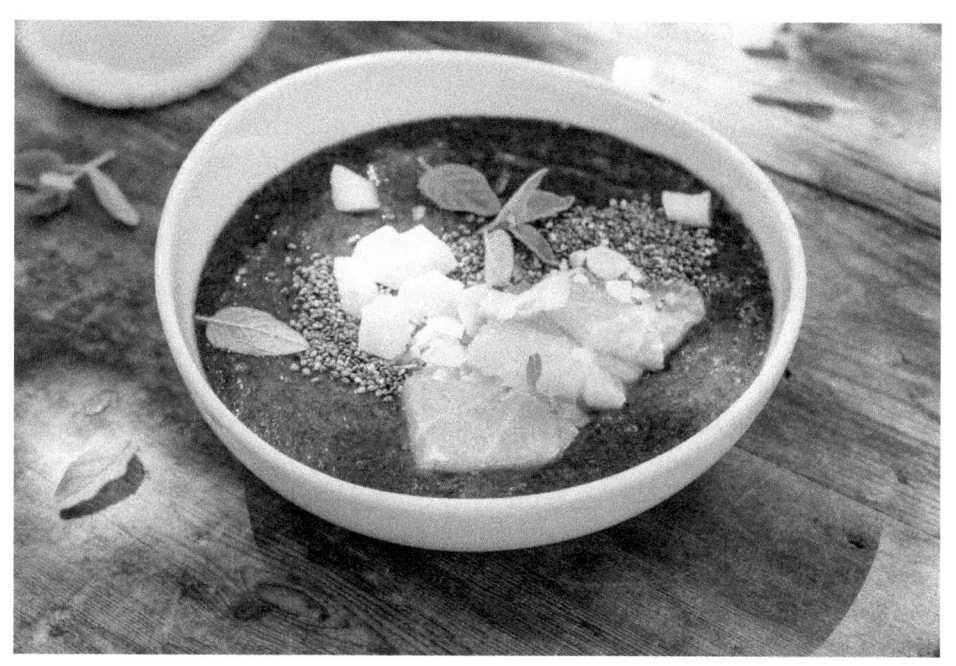

Chickpea Scramble Breakfast Bowl

Serving: 2
Nutrition:
457.5 Cal; 16.3 g Fat; 26.8 g Saturated Fat; 123.5 g Carbohydrates; 39.2 g Fiber; 22.6 g Sugars; 32 g Protein;
Preparation time: 5 minutes
Cooking time: 12 minutes
Ingredients:
For the Chickpea Scramble:
1/4 of a medium white onion, peeled, diced
12 ounces cooked chickpeas
1/2 teaspoon ground black pepper
1/2 teaspoon salt
1/2 teaspoon ground turmeric
1 teaspoon minced garlic
1 teaspoon olive oil
For the Breakfast Bowl:
1 medium avocado, pitted, peeled, diced
1 cup mixed greens
4 tablespoons minced cilantro
4 tablespoons minced parsley
Directions:
Prepare the chickpea scramble and for this, take a large bowl, add chickpeas in it, drizzle with some water and mash with a fork until broken.
Add black pepper, salt, and turmeric into the chickpeas, and then stir until combined.
Take a medium skillet pan, place it over medium heat, add oil and when hot, add onion and cook for 5 minutes until softened. Stir in garlic, continue cooking for 1 minute until fragrant and golden brown, add mashed chickpeas, stir well and cook for 5 minutes or until sauté.

Assemble the bowls and for this, distribute mixed greens evenly between the bowls, top with cooked chickpeas scramble, and then top with parsley and cilantro and avocado slices.
Serve straight away.

Breakfast Grain Salad

Serving: 6
Nutrition:
353 Cal; 20.1 g Fat; 2.5 g Saturated Fat; 38 g Carbohydrates; 5.5 g Fiber; 12.6 g Sugars; 9.3 g Protein;
Preparation time: 40 minutes
Cooking time: 25 minutes
Ingredients:
1 cup golden quinoa
2 cups mixed berries
1/2 cup millet
1 cup oats, steel-cut
1-inch piece of ginger, peeled, sliced into coins
2 lemons, zested, juiced
¾ teaspoon salt
1/2 cup maple syrup
1/4 teaspoon nutmeg
2 cups hazelnuts, chopped, toasted
3 tablespoons olive oil, divided
½ cup of water
1 cup of soy yogurt
Directions:
Take a medium saucepan, about 3-quarts, place it over medium-high heat, add 1 tablespoon oil and when hot, add quinoa, millet, and oats, stir well and cook for 3 minutes until fragrant and toasted.

Add ginger, zest of 1 lemon, salt, and water, stir until mixed and bring the mixture to a boil.

Then switch heat to medium level, simmer for 20 minutes, then remove the pan from heat, cover it with the lid and let it stand for 5 minutes.

After 5 minutes, fluff the grain by using a fork, remove the ginger, transfer grains to a large baking sheet, spread them evenly, and cool for 30 minutes.

Then take a large bowl, transfer cooled grains into it, add the zest of the second lemon and stir until mixed.

Take a medium bowl, add lemon juice and remaining oil and then whisk until emulsified.

Add nutmeg, maple syrup and yogurt, whisk until combined, then pour this mixture into the grains and stir well until coated. Add blueberries and nuts, stir until mixed, taste to adjust seasoning and then serve.

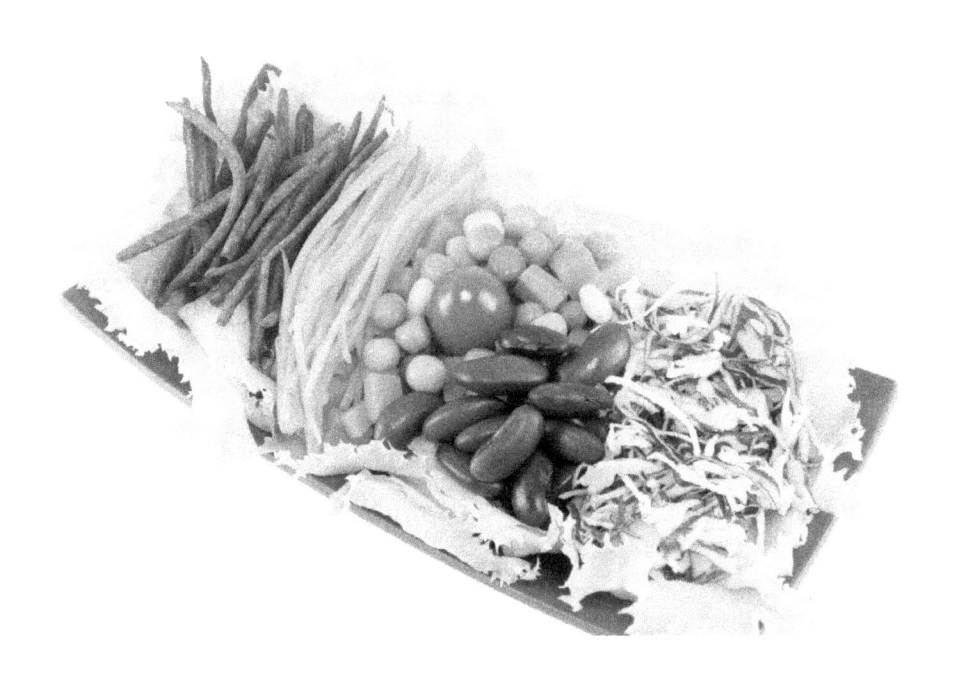

Lunch Recipes

Amazing Potato Dish

Preparation time: 10 minutes
Cooking time: 3 hours
Servings: 4
Ingredients:
1 and ½ pounds potatoes, peeled and roughly chopped
1 tablespoon olive oil
3 tablespoons water
1 small yellow onion, chopped
½ Cup veggie stock cube, crumbled
½ Teaspoon coriander, ground
½ Teaspoon cumin, ground
½ Teaspoon garam masala
½ Teaspoon chili powder
Black pepper to the taste
½ Pound spinach, roughly torn
Directions:
Put the potatoes in your slow cooker.
Add oil, water, onion, stock cube, coriander, cumin, garam masala, chili powder, black pepper and spinach.
Stir, cover and cook on High for 3 hours.
Divide into bowls and serve.
Enjoy!
Nutrition: calories 270, fat 4, fiber 6, carbs 8, protein 12

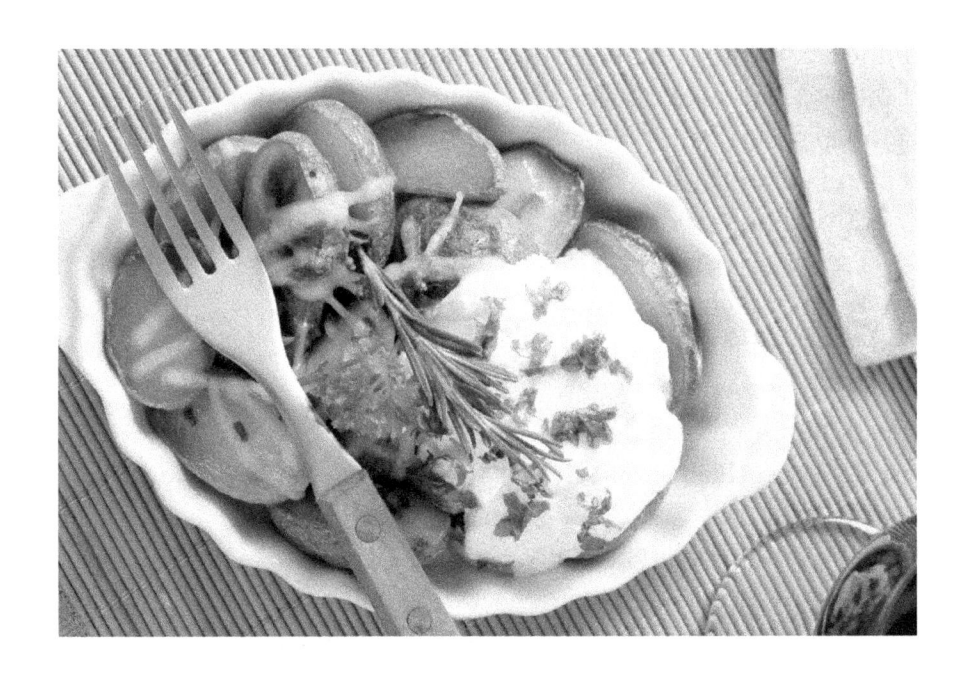

Textured Sweet Potatoes and Lentils Delight

Preparation time: 10 minutes
Cooking time: 4 hours and 30 minutes
Servings: 6
Ingredients:
6 cups sweet potatoes, peeled and cubed
2 teaspoons coriander, ground
2 teaspoons chili powder
1 yellow onion, chopped
3 cups veggie stock
4 garlic cloves, minced
A pinch of sea salt and black pepper
10 ounces canned coconut milk
1 cup water
1 and ½ cups red lentils
Directions:
Put sweet potatoes in your slow cooker.
Add coriander, chili powder, onion, stock, garlic, salt and pepper, stir, cover and cook on high for 3 hours.
Add lentils, stir, cover and cook for 1 hour and 30 minutes.
Add water and coconut milk, stir well, divide into bowls and serve right away.
Enjoy!
Nutrition: calories 300, fat 10, fiber 8, carbs 16, protein 10

Incredibly Tasty Pizza

Preparation time: 1 hour and 10 minutes
Cooking time: 1 hour and 45 minutes
Servings: 3
Ingredients:
For the dough:
½ Teaspoon italian seasoning
1 and ½ cups whole wheat flour
1 and ½ teaspoons instant yeast
1 tablespoon olive oil
A pinch of salt
½ Cup warm water
Cooking spray
For the sauce:
¼ Cup green olives, pitted and sliced
¼ Cup kalamata olives, pitted and sliced
½ Cup tomatoes, crushed
1 tablespoon parsley, chopped
1 tablespoon capers, rinsed
¼ Teaspoon garlic powder
¼ Teaspoon basil, dried
¼ Teaspoon oregano, dried
¼ Teaspoon palm sugar
¼ Teaspoon red pepper flakes
A pinch of salt and black pepper
½ Cup cashew mozzarella, shredded
Directions:
In your food processor, mix yeast with italian seasoning, a pinch of salt and flour.
Add oil and the water and blend well until you obtain a dough. Transfer dough to a floured working surface, knead well, transfer to a greased bowl, cover and leave aside for 1 hour.

Meanwhile, in a bowl, mix green olives with kalamata olives, tomatoes, parsley, capers, garlic powder, oregano, sugar, salt, pepper and pepper flakes and stir well.
Transfer pizza dough to a working surface again and flatten it. Shape so it will fit your slow cooker.
Grease your slow cooker with cooking spray and add dough. Press well on the bottom.
Spread the sauce mix all over, cover and cook on high for 1 hour and 15 minutes.
Spread vegan mozzarella all over, cover again and cook on high for 30 minutes more.
Leave your pizza to cool down before slicing and serving it.
Nutrition: calories 340, fat 5, fiber 7, carbs 13, protein 15

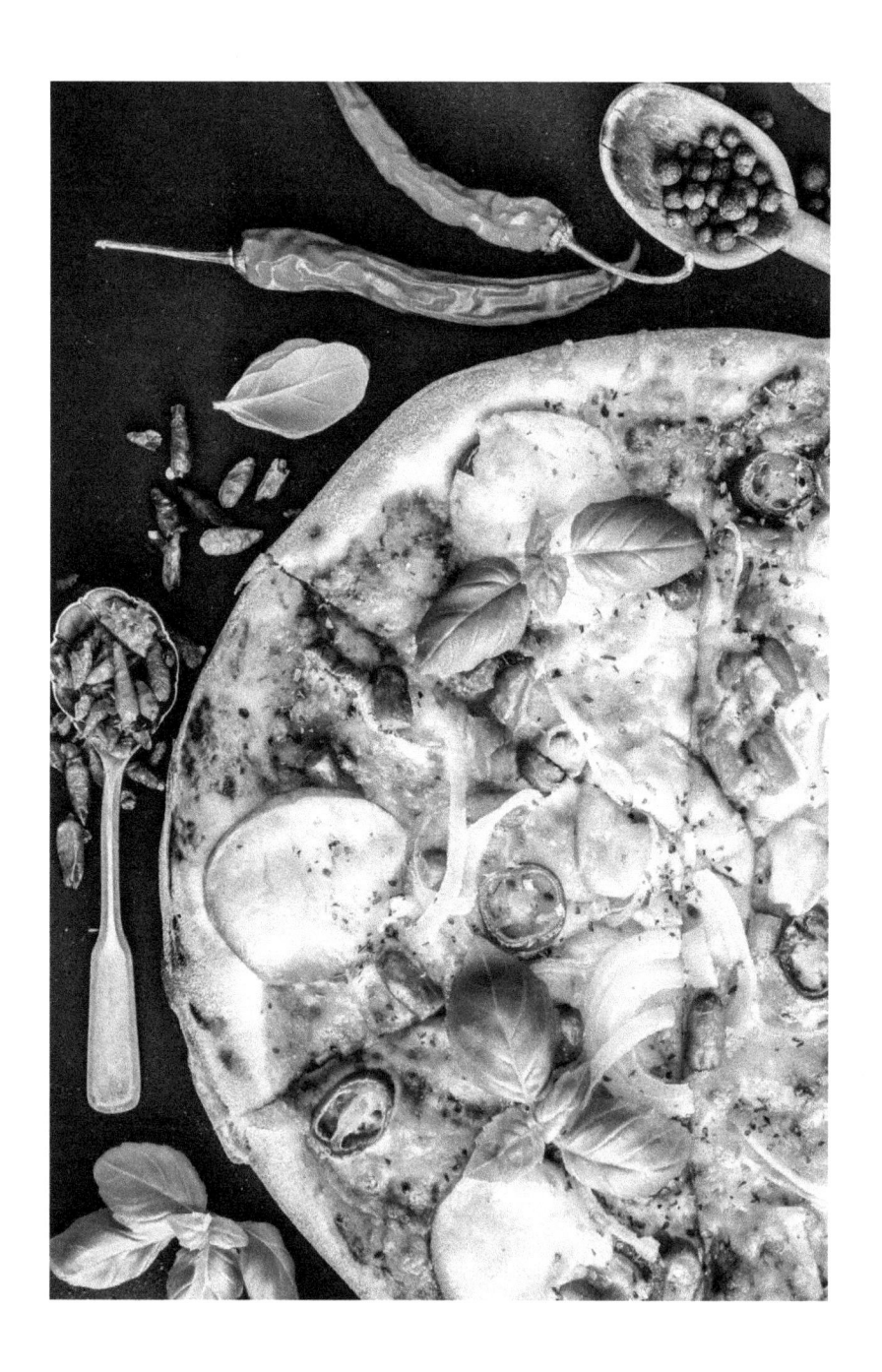

Rich Beans Soup

Preparation time: 10 minutes
Cooking time: 7 hours
Servings: 4
Ingredients:
1 pound navy beans
1 yellow onion, chopped
4 garlic cloves, crushed
2 quarts veggie stock
A pinch of sea salt
Black pepper to the taste
2 potatoes, peeled and cubed
2 teaspoons dill, dried
1 cup sun-dried tomatoes, chopped
1 pound carrots, sliced
4 tablespoons parsley, minced
Directions:
Put the stock in your slow cooker.
Add beans, onion, garlic, potatoes, tomatoes, carrots, dill, salt and pepper, stir, cover and cook on low for 7 hours.
Stir your soup, add parsley, divide into bowls and serve.
Enjoy!
Nutrition: calories 250, fat 4, fiber 3, carbs 9, protein 10

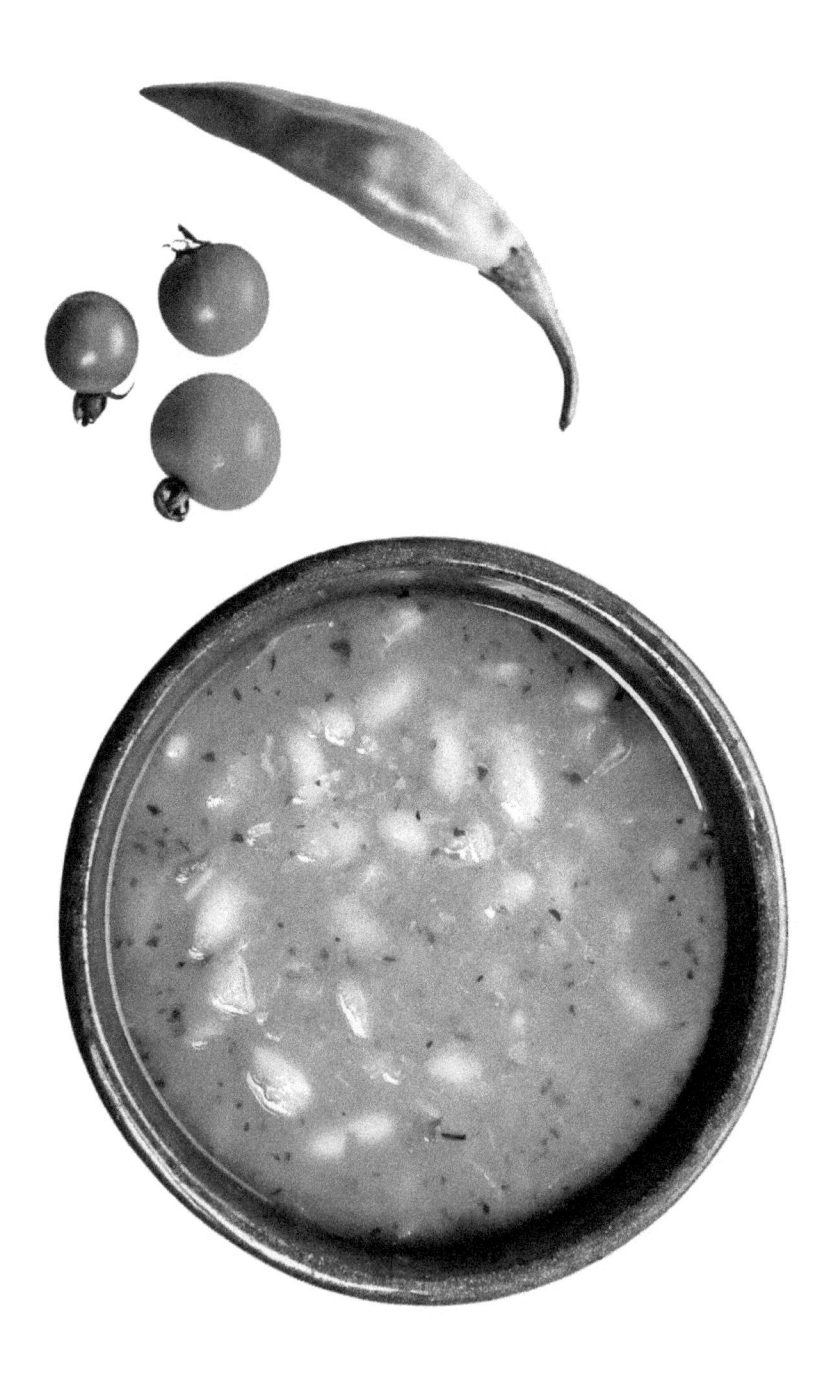

Delicious Baked Beans

Preparation time: 10 minutes
Cooking time: 12 hours
Servings: 8
Ingredients:
1 pound navy beans, soaked overnight and drained
1 cup maple syrup
1 cup bourbon
1 cup vegan bbq sauce
1 cup palm sugar
¼ Cup ketchup
1 cup water
¼ Cup mustard
¼ Cup blackstrap molasses
¼ Cup apple cider vinegar
¼ Cup olive oil
2 tablespoons coconut aminos
Directions:
Put the beans in your slow cooker.
Add maple syrup, bourbon, bbq sauce, sugar, ketchup, water, mustard, molasses, vinegar, oil and coconut aminos.
Stir everything, cover and cook on Low for 12 hours.
Divide into bowls and serve.
Enjoy!
Nutrition: calories 430, fat 7, fiber 8, carbs 15, protein 19

Indian Lentils

Preparation time: 10 minutes
Cooking time: 3 hours
Servings: 4
Ingredients:
1 yellow bell pepper, chopped
1 sweet potato, chopped
2 and ½ cups lentils, already cooked
4 garlic cloves, minced
1 yellow onion, chopped
2 teaspoons cumin, ground
15 ounces canned tomato sauce
½ Teaspoon ginger, ground
A pinch of cayenne pepper
1 tablespoons coriander, ground
1 teaspoon turmeric, ground
2 teaspoons paprika
2/3 cup veggie stock
1 teaspoon garam masala
A pinch of sea salt
Black pepper to the taste
Juice of 1 lemon
Directions:
Put the stock in your slow cooker.
Add potato, lentils, onion, garlic, cumin, bell pepper, tomato sauce, salt, pepper, ginger, coriander, turmeric, paprika, cayenne, garam masala and lemon juice.
Stir, cover and cook on high for 3 hours.
Stir your lentils mix again, divide into bowls and serve.
Enjoy!
Nutrition: calories 300, fat 6, fiber 5, carbs 9, protein 12

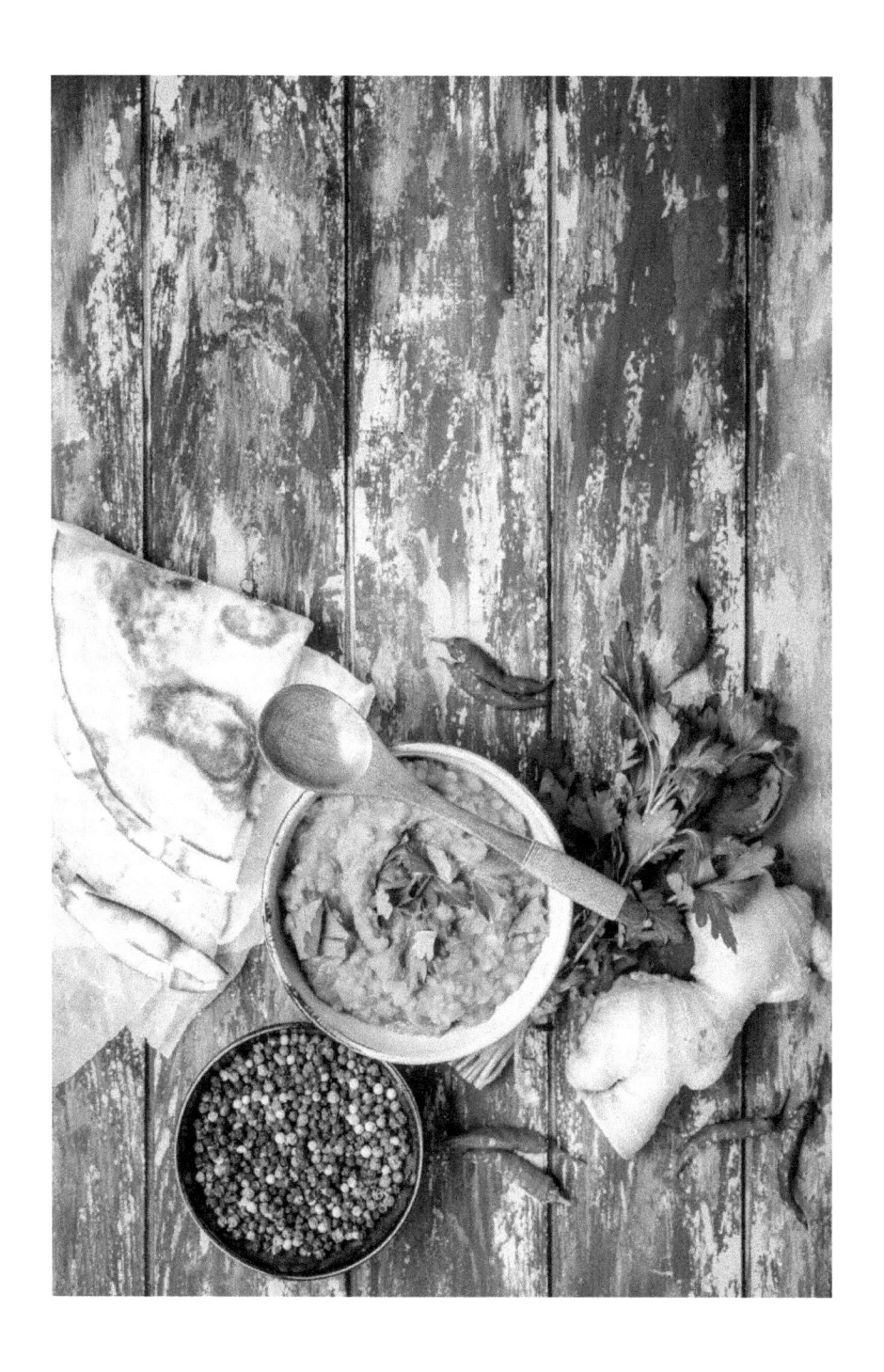

Delicious Butternut Squash Soup

Preparation time: 10 minutes
Cooking time: 6 hours
Servings: 8
Ingredients:
1 apple, cored, peeled and chopped
½ Pound carrots, chopped
1 pound butternut squash, peeled and cubed
1 yellow onion, chopped
A pinch of sea salt
Black pepper to the taste
1 bay leaf
3 cups veggie stock
14 ounces canned coconut milk
¼ Teaspoon sage, dried
Directions:
Put the stock in your slow cooker.
Add apple squash, carrots, onion, salt, pepper and bay leaf.
Stir, cover and cook on low for 6 hours.
Transfer to your blender, add coconut milk and sage and pulse really well.
Ladle into bowls and serve right away.
Enjoy!
Nutrition: calories 200, fat 3, fiber 6, carbs 8, protein 10

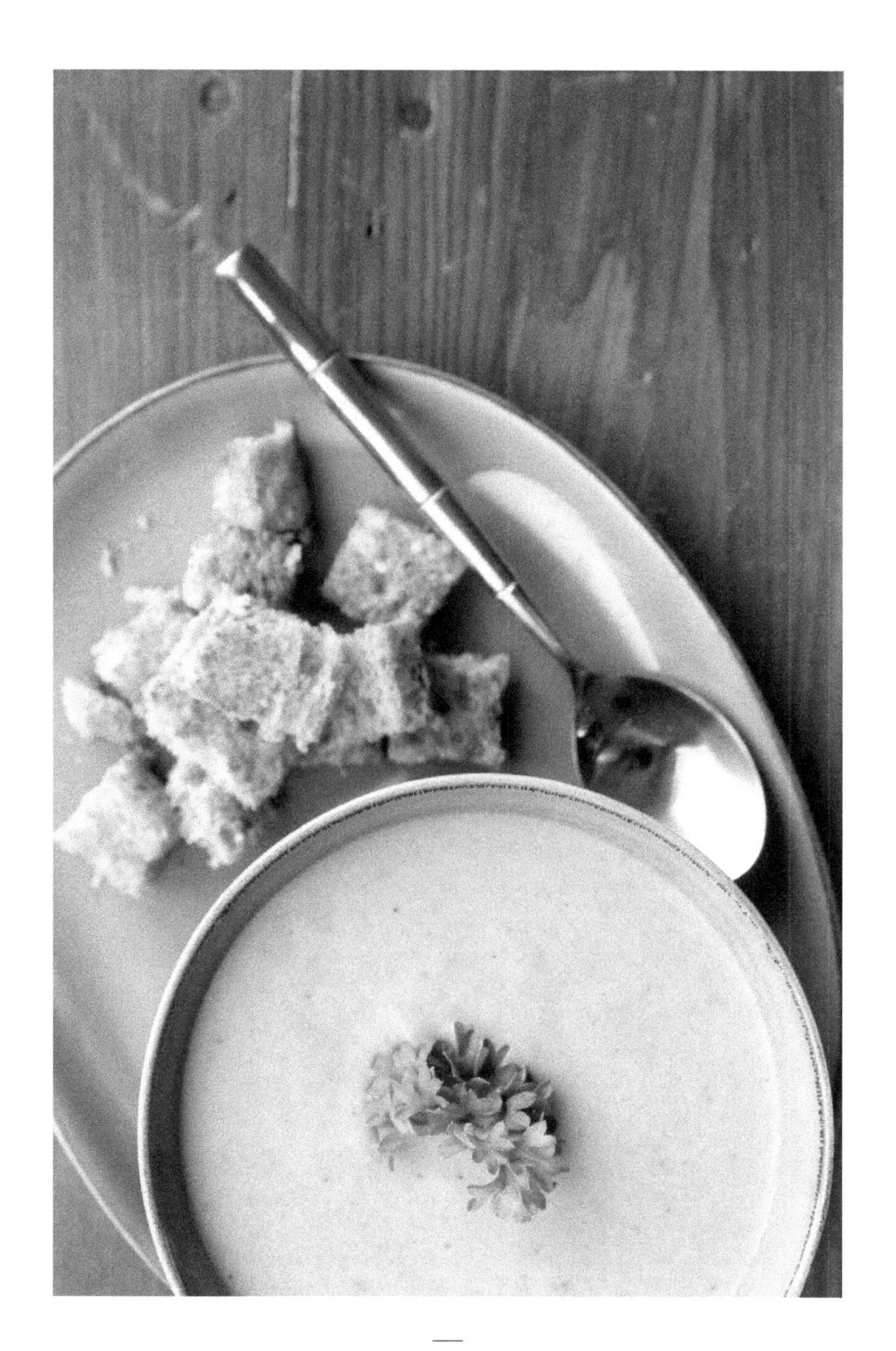

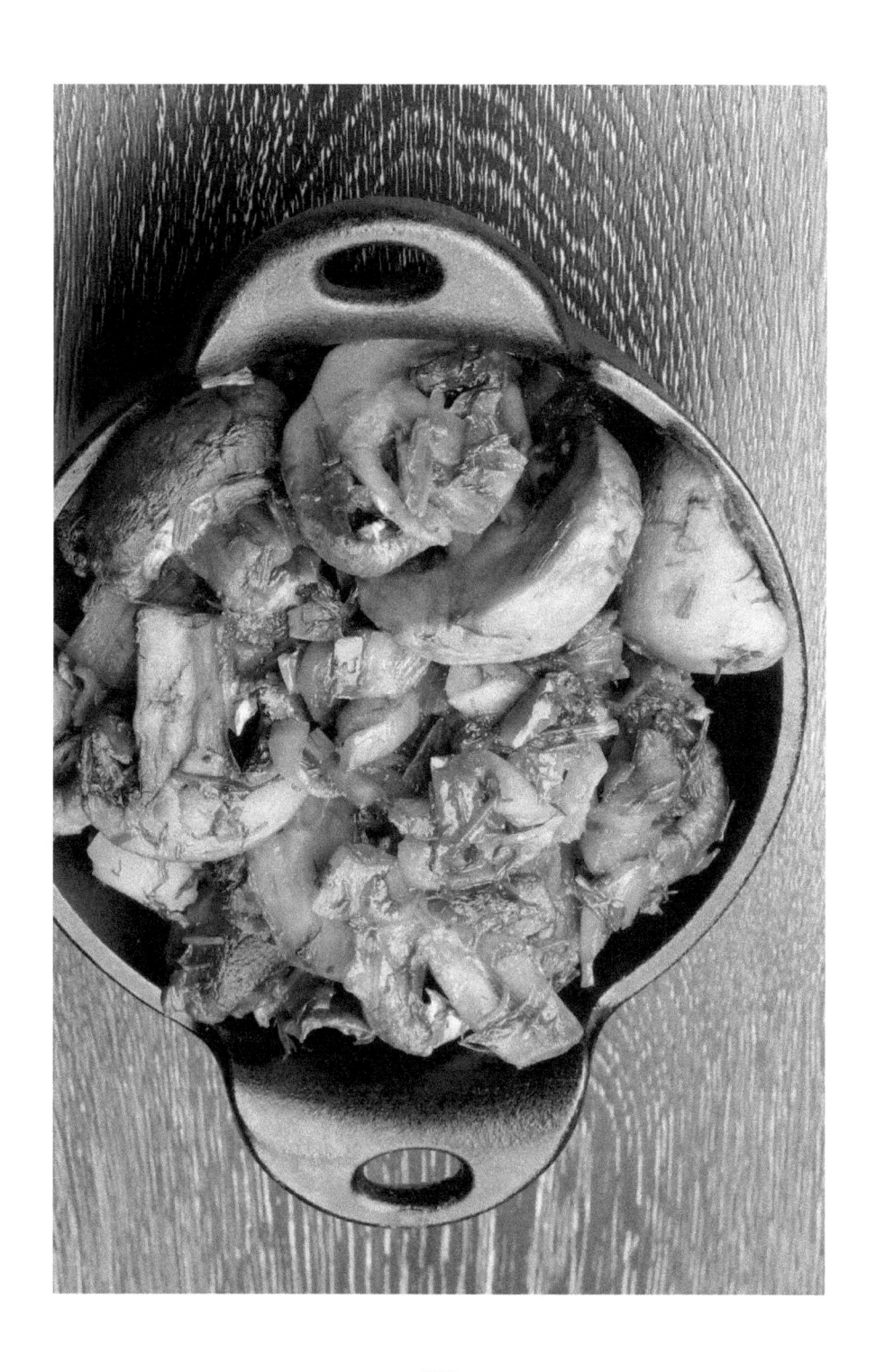

Amazing Mushroom Stew

Preparation time: 10 minutes
Cooking time: 8 hours
Servings: 4
Ingredients:
2 garlic cloves, minced
1 celery stalk, chopped
1 yellow onion, chopped
1 and ½ cups firm tofu, pressed and cubed
1 cup water
10 ounces mushrooms, chopped
1 pound mixed peas, corn and carrots
2 and ½ cups veggie stock
1 teaspoon thyme, dried
2 tablespoons coconut flour
A pinch of sea salt
Black pepper to the taste
Directions:
Put the water and stock in your slow cooker.
Add garlic, onion, celery, mushrooms, mixed veggies, tofu, thyme, salt, pepper and flour.
Stir everything, cover and cook on low for 8 hours.
Divide into bowls and serve hot.
Enjoy!
Nutrition: calories 230, fat 4, fiber 6, carbs 10, protein 7

Simple Tofu Dish

Preparation time: 10 minutes
Cooking time: 3 hours
Servings: 6
Ingredients:
1 big tofu package, cubed
1 tablespoon sesame oil
¼ Cup pineapple, cubed
1 tablespoon olive oil
2 garlic cloves, minced
1 tablespoons brown rice vinegar
2 teaspoon ginger, grated
¼ Cup soy sauce
5 big zucchinis, cubed
¼ Cup sesame seeds
Directions:
In your food processor, mix sesame oil with pineapple, olive oil, garlic, ginger, soy sauce and vinegar and whisk well.
Add this to your slow cooker and mix with tofu cubes.
Cover and cook on High for 2 hours and 45 minutes.
Add sesame seeds and zucchinis, stir gently, cover and cook on High for 15 minutes.
Divide between plates and serve.
Enjoy!
Nutrition: calories 200, fat 3, fiber 4, carbs 9, protein 10

Special Jambalaya

Preparation time: 10 minutes
Cooking time: 6 hours
Servings: 4
Ingredients:
6 ounces soy chorizo, chopped
1 and ½ cups celery ribs, chopped
1 cup okra
1 green bell pepper, chopped
16 ounces canned tomatoes and green chilies, chopped
2 garlic cloves, minced
½ Teaspoon paprika
1 and ½ cups veggie stock
A pinch of cayenne pepper
Black pepper to the taste
A pinch of salt
3 cups already cooked wild rice for serving
Directions:
Heat up a pan over medium high heat, add soy chorizo, stir, brown for a few minutes and transfer to your slow cooker.
Also, add celery, bell pepper, okra, tomatoes and chilies, garlic, paprika, salt, pepper and cayenne to your slow cooker.
Stir everything, add veggie stock, cover the slow cooker and cook on low for 6 hours.
Divide rice on plates, top each serving with your vegan jambalaya and serve hot.
Enjoy!
Nutrition: calories 150, fat 3, fiber 7, carbs 15, protein 9

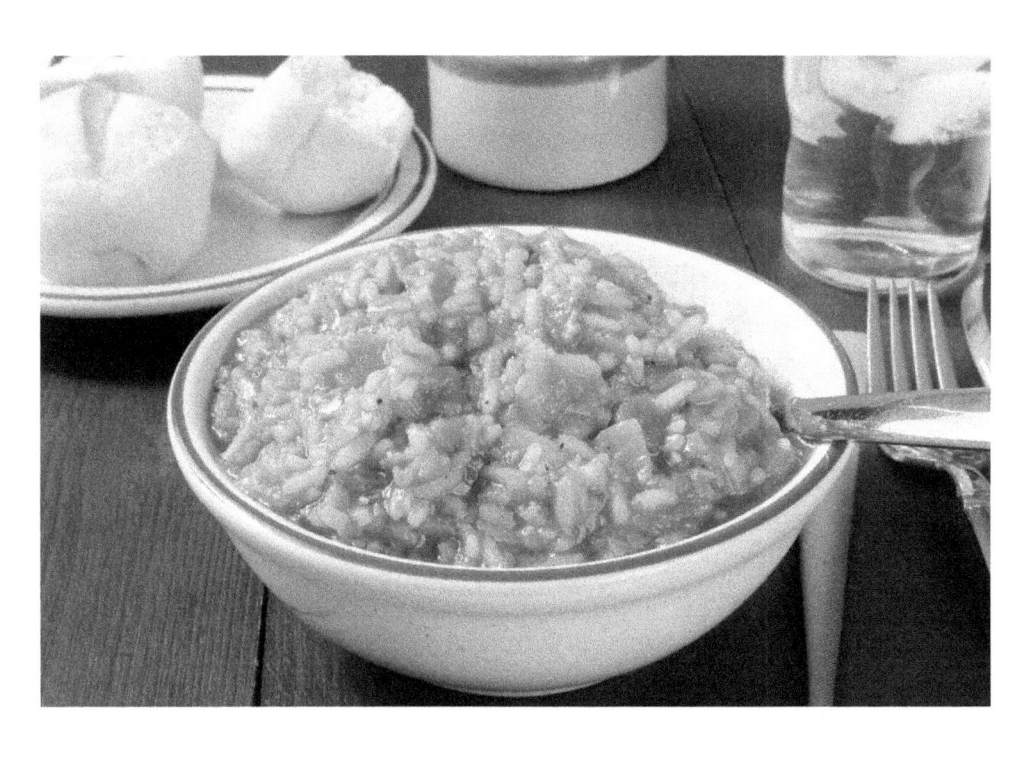

Delicious Chard Soup

Preparation time: 10 minutes
Cooking time: 8 hours
Servings: 6
Ingredients:
1 yellow onion, chopped
1 tablespoon olive oil
1 celery stalk, chopped
2 garlic cloves, minced
1 carrot, chopped
1 bunch swiss chard, torn
1 cup brown lentils, dried
5 potatoes, peeled and cubed
1 tablespoon soy sauce
Black pepper to the taste
A pinch of sea salt
6 cups veggie stock
Directions:
Heat up a big pan with the oil over medium high heat, add onion, celery, garlic, carrot and Swiss chard, stir, cook for a few minutes and transfer to your slow cooker.
Also, add lentils, potatoes, soy sauce, salt, pepper and stock to the slow cooker, stir, cover and cook on Low for 8 hours.
Divide into bowls and serve hot.
Enjoy!
Nutrition: calories 200, fat 4, fiber 5, carbs 9, protein 12

Chinese Tofu and Veggies

Preparation time: 10 minutes
Cooking time: 4 hours
Servings: 4
Ingredients:
14 ounces extra firm tofu, pressed and cut into medium triangles
Cooking spray
2 teaspoons ginger, grated
1 yellow onion, chopped
3 garlic cloves, minced
8 ounces tomato sauce
¼ Cup hoisin sauce
¼ Teaspoon coconut aminos
2 tablespoons rice wine vinegar
1 tablespoon soy sauce
1 tablespoon spicy mustard
¼ Teaspoon red pepper, crushed
2 teaspoons molasses
2 tablespoons water
A pinch of black pepper
3 broccoli stalks
1 green bell pepper, cut into squares
2 zucchinis, cubed
Directions:
Heat up a pan over medium high heat, add tofu pieces, brown them for a few minutes and transfer to your slow cooker.
Heat up the pan again over medium high heat, add ginger, onion, garlic and tomato sauce, stir, sauté for a few minutes and transfer to your slow cooker as well.
Add hoisin sauce, aminos, vinegar, soy sauce, mustard, red pepper, molasses, water and black pepper, stir gently, cover and cook on high for 3 hours.

Add zucchinis, bell pepper and broccoli, cover and cook on high for 1 more hour.
Divide between plates and serve right away.
Enjoy!
Nutrition: calories 300, fat 4, fiber 8, carbs 14, protein 13

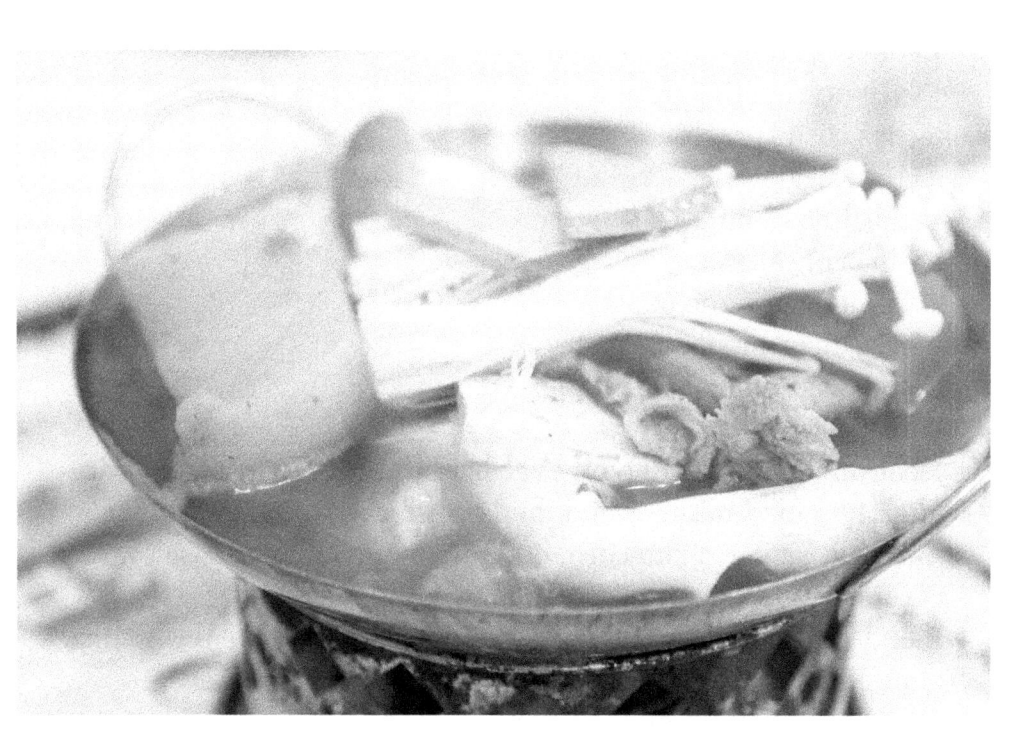

Wonderful Corn Chowder

Preparation time: 10 minutes
Cooking time: 8 hours and 30 minutes
Servings: 6
Ingredients:
2 cups yellow onion, chopped
2 tablespoons olive oil
1 red bell pepper, chopped
1 pound gold potatoes, cubed
1 teaspoon cumin, ground
4 cups corn kernels
4 cups veggie stock
1 cup almond milk
A pinch of salt
A pinch of cayenne pepper
½ Teaspoon smoked paprika
Chopped scallions for serving
Directions:
Heat up a pan with the oil over medium heat, add onion, stir and sauté for 5 minutes and then transfer to your slow cooker.
Add bell pepper, 1 cup corn, potatoes, paprika, cumin, salt and cayenne, stir, cover and cook on low for 8 hours.
Blend this using an immersion blender and then mix with almond milk and the rest of the corn.
Stir chowder, cover and cook on low for 30 minutes more.
Ladle into bowls and serve with chopped scallions on top.
Enjoy!
Nutrition: calories 200, fat 4, fiber 7, carbs 13, protein 16

Black Eyed Peas Stew

Preparation time: 10 minutes
Cooking time: 4 hours
Servings: 8
Ingredients:
3 celery stalks, chopped
2 carrots, sliced
1 yellow onion, chopped
1 sweet potato, cubed
1 green bell pepper, chopped
3 cups black-eyed peas, soaked for 8 hours and drained
1 cup tomato puree
4 cups veggie stock
A pinch of salt
Black pepper to the taste
1 chipotle chile, minced
1 teaspoon ancho chili powder
1 teaspoons sage, dried and crumbled
2 teaspoons cumin, ground
Chopped coriander for serving
Directions:
Put celery in your slow cooker.
Add carrots, onion, potato, bell pepper, black-eyed peas, tomato puree, salt, pepper, chili powder, sage, chili, cumin and stock.
Stir, cover and cook on High for 4 hours.
Stir stew again, divide into bowls and serve with chopped coriander on top.
Enjoy!
Nutrition: calories 200, fat 4, fiber 7, carbs 9, protein 16

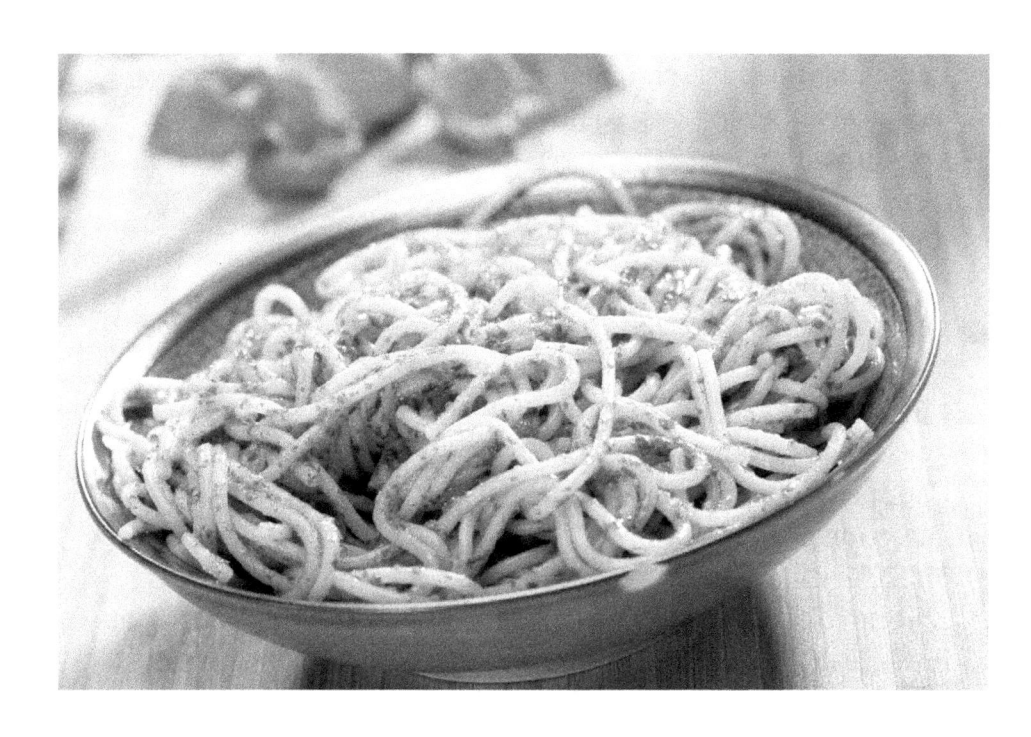

Dinner Recipes

Pesto Spaghetti with Chickpea Balls

Serving: 4
Nutrition:
636 Cal; 21.8 g Fat; 2 g Saturated Fat; 88 g Carbohydrates; 14 g Fiber; 9 g Sugars; 24 g Protein;
Preparation time: 10 minutes
Cooking time: 40 minutes
Ingredients:
For the Chickpea Meatballs:
1/3 cup walnuts
1 1/2 cups cooked chickpeas
1 small white onion, peeled, chopped
¼ cup basil leaves
1 1/2 tablespoon minced garlic
1/4 cup breadcrumbs
2 tablespoons flax meal
1/4 teaspoon red pepper flakes
1/2 teaspoon salt
2 tablespoons nutritional yeast
1 teaspoon oregano
1/2 teaspoon chopped parsley
1 tablespoon olive oil
1/4 cup water
For the Pesto:
2 cups basil leaves
1 teaspoon minced garlic
1 tablespoon nutritional yeast
2 tablespoons walnuts
1/4 teaspoon salt

1 tablespoon lemon juice
1 tablespoon olive oil
2 tablespoons water
For the Pasta:
8 ounces of spaghetti, whole-wheat, cooked
½ teaspoon cracked black pepper, for garnish
Directions:
Prepare the pesto and for this, place basil in a food processor, add nuts, garlic, and yeast and pulse for 2 minutes until minced. Add salt, lemon juice, water, and oil, blend for 1 minute until smooth, then tip the mixture in a bowl and set aside until required.

Prepare the chickpea balls and for this, take a medium skillet pan, add ½ teaspoon oil and when hot, add onion and garlic and cook for 4 minutes until softened.

Place nuts in a food processor, pulse for 1 minute until ground, add onion mixture along with remaining ingredients for the meatballs except for breadcrumbs, and then pulse for 2 minutes until combined.

Transfer the chickpea mixture into a bowl, add breadcrumbs, stir until mixed, and then chill the mixture for 10 minutes.

Meanwhile, switch on the oven, then set it to 425 degrees F and let it preheat.

After 10 minutes, shape the chickpea mixture into small balls, about 1 ½-inch thick, arrange them on a baking sheet lined with parchment and bake for 25 minutes until golden.

Meanwhile, take a medium pot half full with water, place it over medium heat, bring it to a boil, add spaghetti, cook for 7 to 10 minutes until tender, and, when done, drain the spaghetti and set aside until required.

When meatballs have cooked, transfer them to the ball containing pesto and toss until well coated.

Distribute pasta among plates, top with the chickpea balls, sprinkle cracked black pepper on top and then serve.

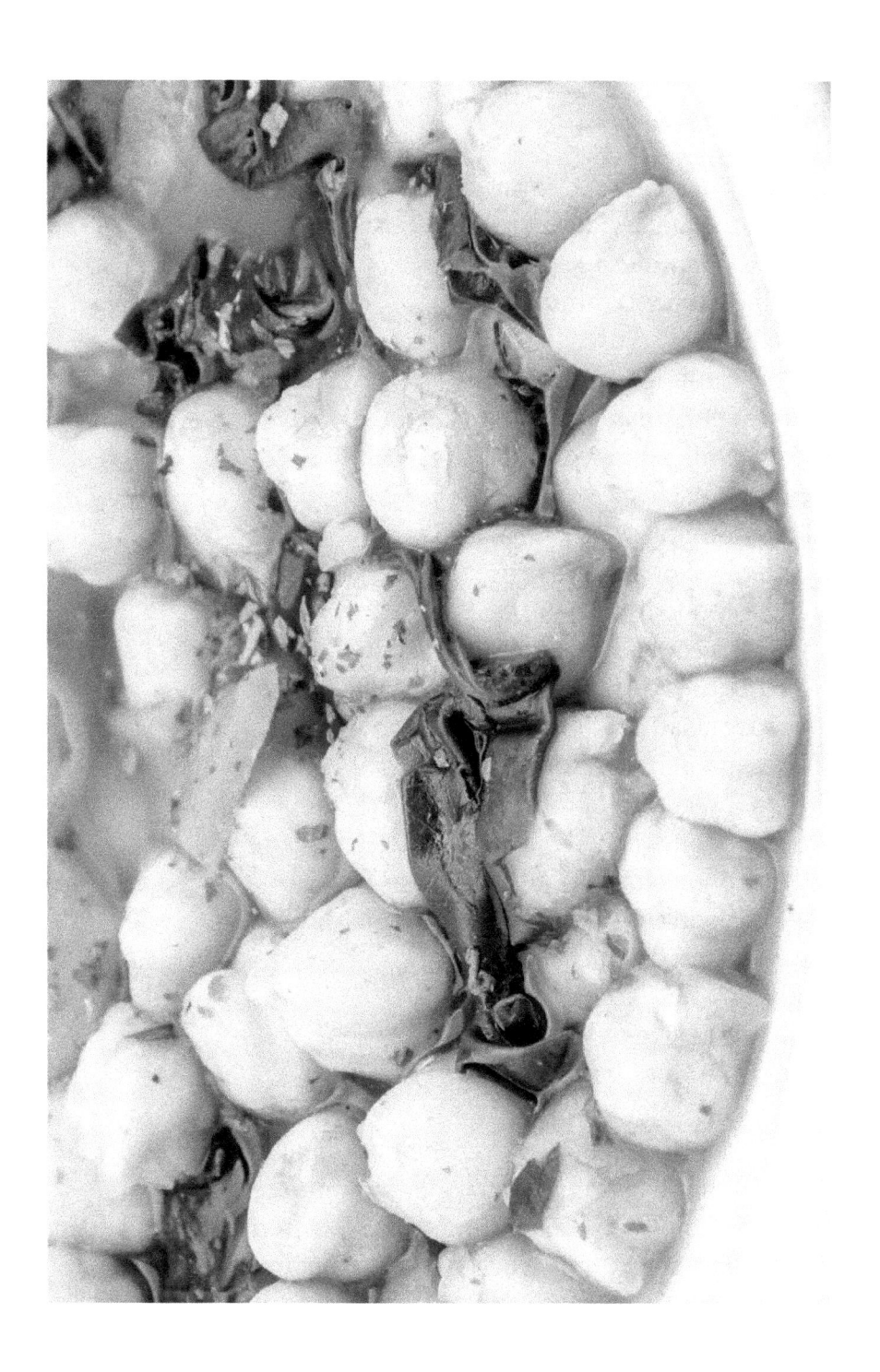

Chickpea, Quinoa and Spinach Stew

Serving: 3
Nutrition:
423 Cal; 9 g Fat; 1 g Saturated Fat; 66 g Carbohydrates; 18 g Fiber; 10 g Sugars; 21 g Protein;
Preparation time: 10 minutes
Cooking time: 30 minutes
Ingredients:
1/2 cup chopped red onion
1 tablespoon minced garlic
1 green chili, chopped
2 cups spinach
2 large tomatoes
1-inch piece of ginger
1/4 cup red lentils
1 1/2 cups cooked chickpeas
1/4 cup quinoa
1 teaspoon salt
1/4 teaspoon cinnamon powder
1 teaspoon garam masala
1/4 teaspoon cracked black pepper
1/2 teaspoon cumin powder
1/4 teaspoon cardamom powder
1/2 teaspoon coconut sugar
2 tablespoons chopped cashews
1 teaspoon olive oil
2 cups of water
Directions:
Take a large pot, place it over medium heat, add oil and when hot, add onion and chili and cook for 5 minutes.
Meanwhile, place spinach and tomatoes in a food processor, add ginger, garlic, and black pepper, pour in ½ cup water and pulse for 2 minutes until smooth.

Add all the spices, stir well, cook for 1 minute, pour in tomato puree, add chickpeas, lentils, and quinoa, season with salt and sugar, pour in the remaining water, stir until mixed and cook for 20 minutes until thoroughly cooked.

Then add cashew, taste the stew to adjust seasoning, and cook for 3 minutes.

Serve straight away.

Tofu Soba Noodles

Serving: 4
Nutrition:
383.5 Cal; 12 g Fat; 5.7 g Saturated Fat; 53 g Carbohydrates; 5 g Fiber; 2 g Sugars; 18.7 g Protein;
Preparation time: 10 minutes
Cooking time: 10 minutes
Ingredients:
1 pound soba noodles, cooked
14 ounces tofu, firm, cubed
2 green onions, thinly sliced
2 cups shredded cabbage
½ teaspoon minced garlic
1 teaspoon grated ginger
1 teaspoon sesame seeds
2 teaspoons brown sugar
1/4 cup rice vinegar
1 tablespoon sesame oil
2 tablespoons soy sauce
1 tablespoon olive oil
2 tablespoons crushed peanuts, for serving
2 tablespoons Sriracha, for serving
Directions:
Prepare the sauce and for this, take a medium bowl, add sesame oil and seeds along with sugar, vinegar, and soy sauce and whisk until combined.
Take a large skillet pan, place it over medium-high heat, add oil and when hot, add tofu pieces and cook for 5 minutes until golden brown.
Transfer the tofu pieces to a plate, add cabbage, ginger, and garlic, stir until mixed, and then cook for 2 minutes until tender.

Then take a large bowl, place cooked soba noodles in it, drizzle with the sauce, add cooked cabbage, green onion, and tofu pieces and toss until mixed.

Garnish noodles with peanuts and Sriracha sauce and then serve.

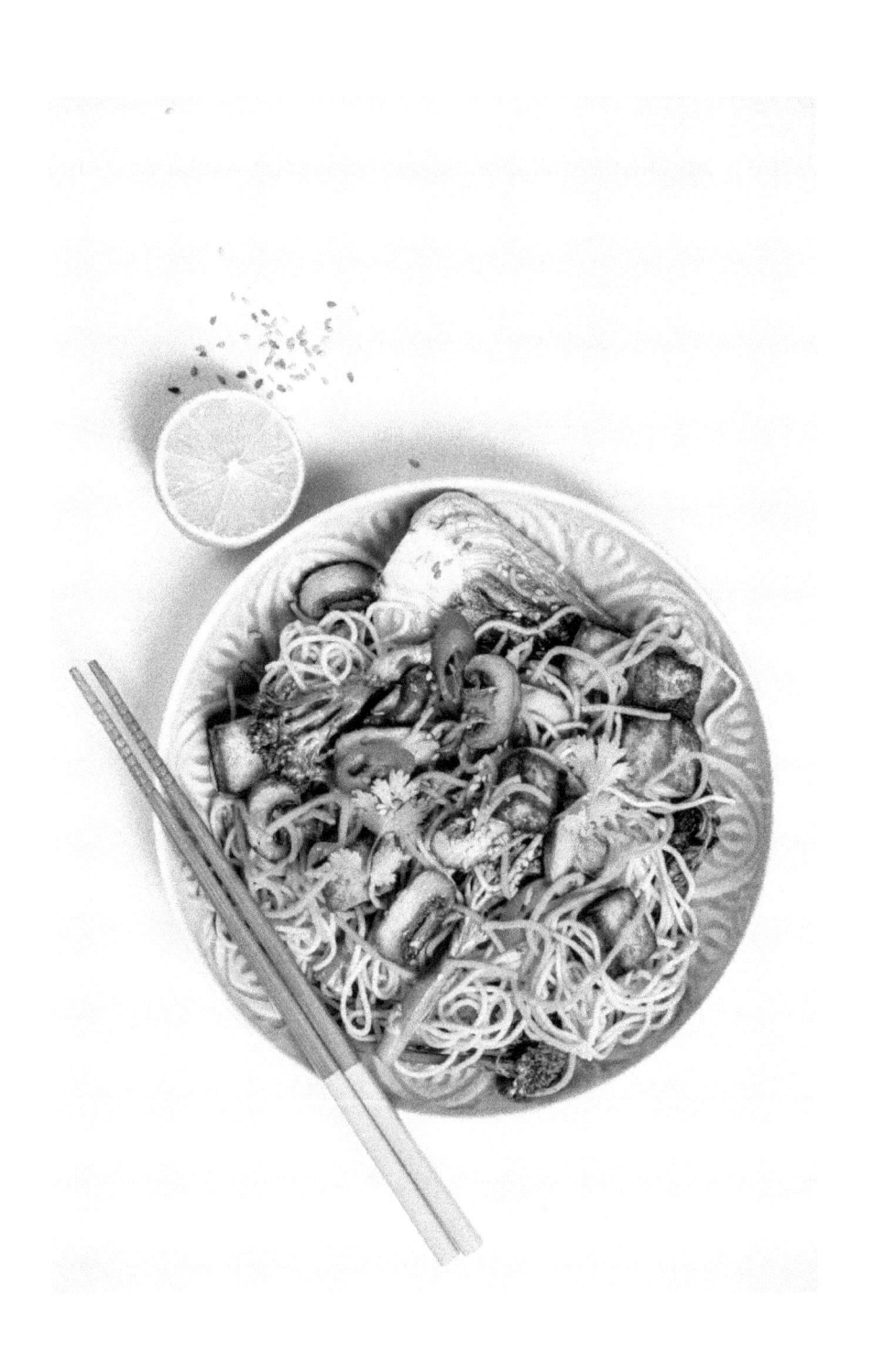

Buffalo Cauliflower Tacos

Serving: 4
Nutrition:
508 Cal; 17.7 g Fat; 3 g Saturated Fat; 76.2 g Carbohydrates; 10.8 g Fiber; 9.1 g Sugars; 15.5 g Protein;
Preparation time: 10 minutes
Cooking time: 30 minutes
Ingredients:
For the Buffalo Cauliflower Tacos:
1 cup all-purpose flour
1 cup almond milk, unsweetened
1/4 teaspoon garlic powder
1/4 teaspoon salt
1/4 teaspoon ground black pepper
5 cups cauliflower florets
3/4 cup hot sauce
2 cups shredded cabbage
1 cup chopped cilantro
8 corn tortillas
For the Avocado Cream:
2 medium avocados, pitted
1/2 teaspoon salt
½ teaspoon minced garlic
2 tablespoons lime juice
1/4 cup vegan sour cream
1/4 cup water
Directions:
Prepare the cauliflower and for this, switch on the oven, then set it to 450 degrees F and let it preheat.
Meanwhile, take a medium bowl, add flour in it along with garlic powder, black pepper, and salt, pour in the milk, and whisk until smooth.

Dip each cauliflower florets into the flour mixture until evenly coated, arrange them on a baking sheet lined with parchment paper and then bake for 20 minutes until browned and crisp.

When done, take a large bowl, place hot sauce in it, add roasted cauliflower florets, toss until coated, return the florets into the oven and continue baking for 10 minutes until glazed.

Meanwhile, prepare the avocado cream and for this, place all of its ingredients in a food processor and then pulse for 2 minutes until smooth.

Distribute cauliflower florets among tortillas, top with cabbage and cilantro, drizzle with prepared avocado cream and then serve.

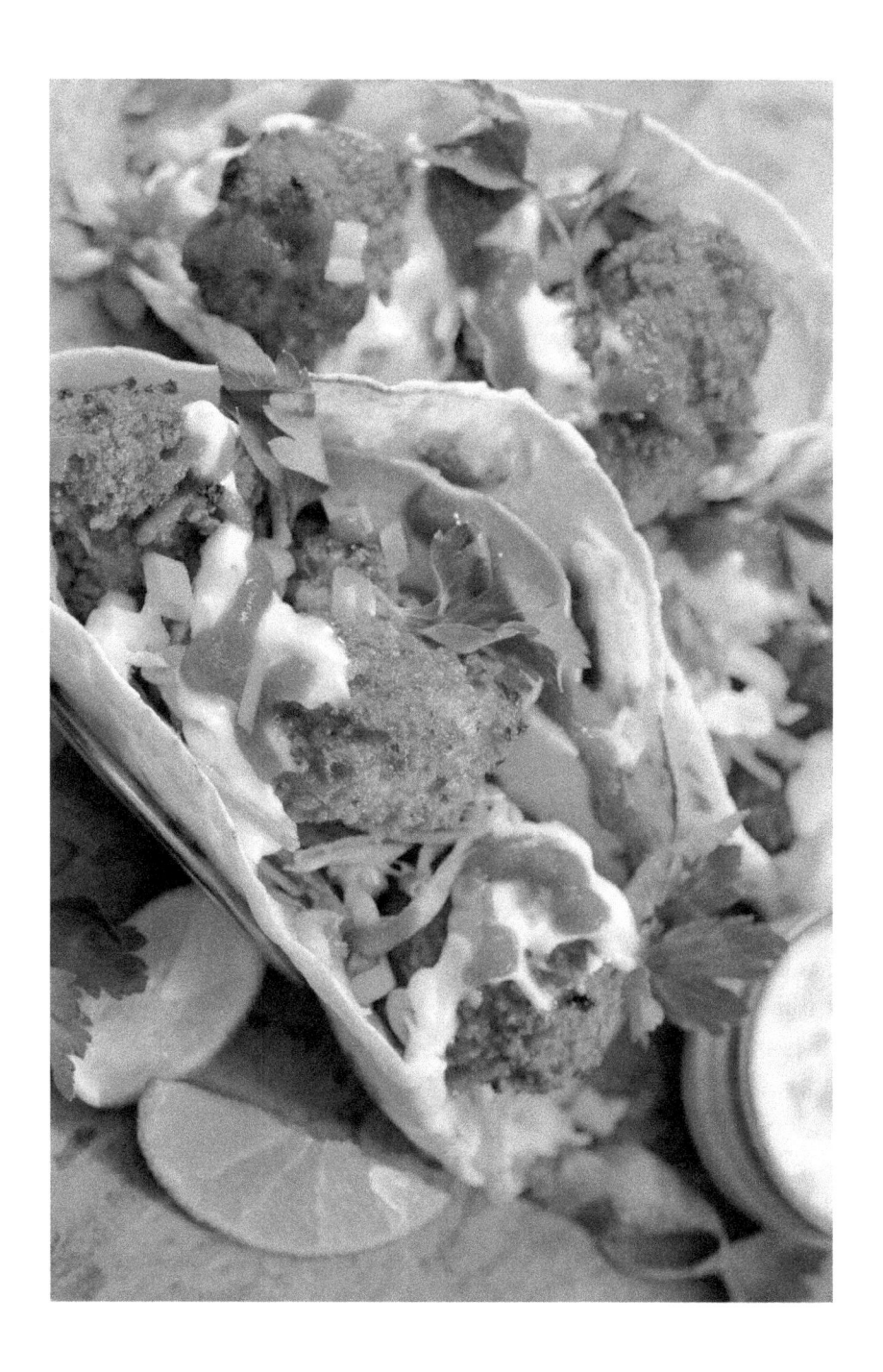

Tofu Steaks with Salad

Serving: 4
Nutrition:
198 Cal; 6.5 g Fat; 1 g Saturated Fat; 19 g Carbohydrates; 6 g Fiber; 3 g Sugars; 12 g Protein;
Preparation time: 1 hour and 10 minutes
Cooking time: 6 minutes
Ingredients:
For the Salad:
2 green shallots, chopped
20 ounces tofu, firm,
1/2 teaspoon grated ginger
½ teaspoon minced garlic
2 tablespoons soy sauce
1 teaspoon wasabi paste
2 teaspoons sesame seeds
For the Salad:
¼ cup snow pea sprouts ends trimmed
1 bunch of rocket, leaves torn into small pieces
5 green shallots, cut into strips
1 nori sheet, halved, shredded crossway
½ teaspoon minced garlic
1 teaspoon caster sugar
¼ teaspoon ground black pepper
1 tablespoon white vinegar
1/4 teaspoon wasabi paste
2 teaspoons soy sauce
Directions:
Prepare the tofu and for this, cut tofu into ½-inch thick slices and then place them in a large bowl.
Take a small bowl, place shallots in it, add sesame seeds, shallots, ginger, garlic, soy sauce, and wasabi and stir until well mixed.

Drizzle this mixture over tofu slices, then turn until well coated and marinate for a minimum of 1 hour at room temperature.

Meanwhile, prepare the salad and for this, take a large salad bowl, add shallots, sprouts, rockets, and nori sheets and set aside until required.

Prepare the drizzle for this, take a small bowl, add garlic, wasabi, black pepper, sugar, soy sauce, and vinegar, whisk until combined, and set aside until required.

When tofu has marinated, take a large frying pan, place it over medium heat, place tofu slices in it and cook for 3 minutes per side until golden.

Transfer tofu pieces to a plate, top with prepared salad, then drizzle with dressing and serve.

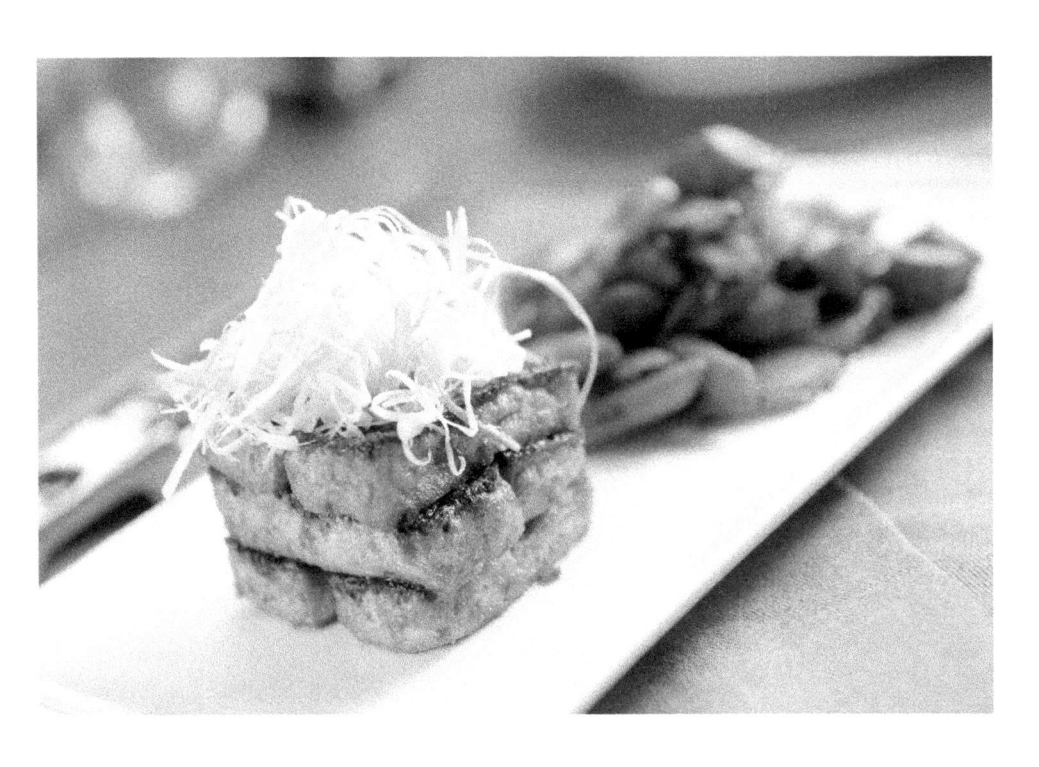

Spinach Ricotta Lasagna

Serving: 6
Nutrition:
300 Cal; 12 g Fat; 6 g Saturated Fat; 26 g Carbohydrates; 3 g Fiber; 6 g Sugars; 24 g Protein;
Preparation time: 10 minutes
Cooking time: 50 minutes
Ingredients:
For the Ricotta Filling:
18 ounces tofu, extra-firm, pressed, cubed
5 cloves of garlic, peeled
2 lemons, juiced
¼ teaspoon ground black pepper
½ teaspoon salt
¼ teaspoon nutmeg
1 tablespoon mustard
2 tablespoons olive oil
For the Sauce:
¼ cup all-purpose flour
½ teaspoon salt
¼ cup almond butter
3 cups of soy milk
For the Tomato sauce:
¾ cup passata
18 ounces frozen spinach, thawed, drained
¼ teaspoon ground black pepper
1/3 teaspoon salt
2 teaspoons dried oregano
8.8 ounces lasagna sheets
Directions:
Prepare the ricotta filling and for this, place all of its ingredients in a food processor except for tofu pieces and then pulse for 2 minutes until smooth.

Add tofu pieces, continue blending for 1 minute until smooth, tip the filling in a medium bowl, and set aside until required.

Prepare the sauce and for this, take a small saucepan, place it over medium heat, add butter and flour and cook for 5 minutes until the thick paste comes together, stirring continuously.

Then whisk in salt and milk, cook for 2 minutes until the sauce has thickened and set aside until required.

Prepare the tomato sauce and for this, take a medium bowl, add passata in it, season with black pepper, salt, and oregano, stir until mixed and set aside until required.

Assemble the lasagna and for this, take a baking dish, layer it bottoms with some lasagna sheets, layer with some spinach, ricotta filling, sauce, and tomato sauce and continue creating more layers, covering the top layer with tomato.

Bake the lasagna for 40 minutes until thoroughly cooked, then cut it into wedges and serve.

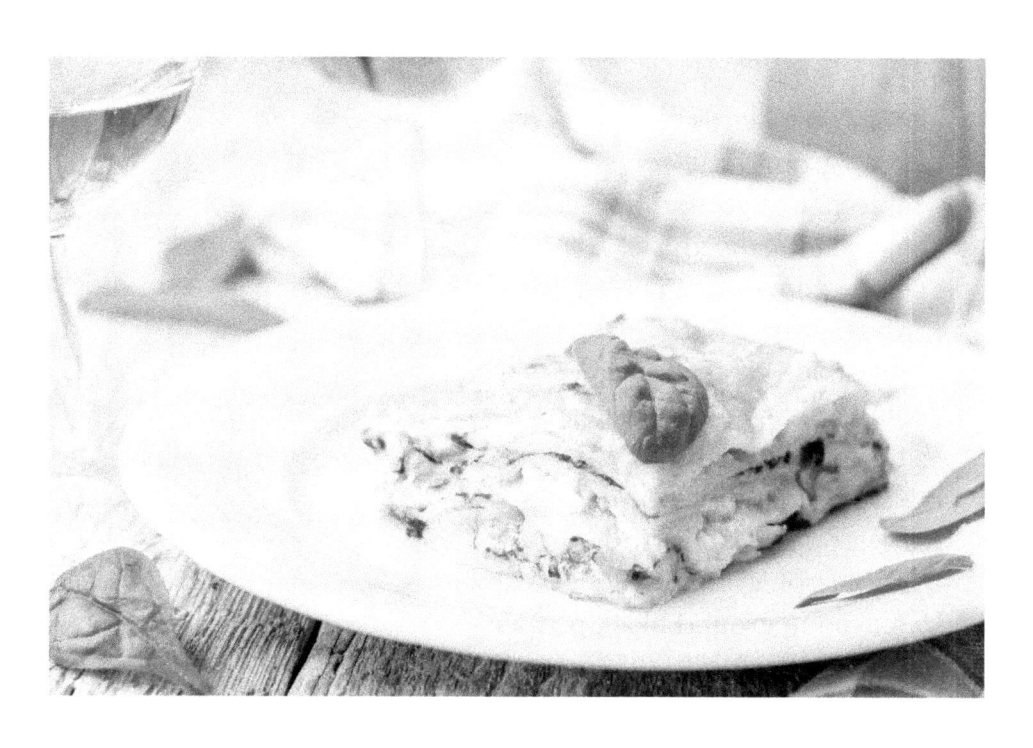

Lentil Loaf

Serving: 8
Nutrition:
259 Cal; 2 g Fat; 0.6 g Saturated Fat; 46 g Carbohydrates; 8 g Fiber; 5.4 g Sugars; 11.3 g Protein;
Preparation time: 15 minutes
Cooking time: 1 hour and 30 minutes
Ingredients:
For the Loaf:
3/4 cup oats
1 cup brown lentils
1/2 cup ground oats
3 tablespoons ground flaxseeds
1 celery stalk, diced
1 small white onion, peeled, diced
1 carrot, grated
1 tablespoon minced garlic
1 small red bell pepper, diced
½ teaspoon of sea salt
1/2 teaspoon onion powder
1/2 teaspoon garlic powder
1/2 teaspoon ground chipotle pepper
½ teaspoon ground black pepper
1/2 teaspoon cumin
1 teaspoon dried thyme
2 1/2 cups vegetable broth
2 tablespoons olive oil
1/3 cup water
For the Glaze:
1 tablespoon maple syrup
1 tablespoon balsamic vinegar
3 tablespoons ketchup
Directions:

Cook the lentils and for this, take a large pot, place it over medium-high heat, add lentils, pour in 2 ½ cups water, and bring it to a boil.

Switch heat to medium-low level and then simmer for 40 minutes until tender, covering the pot.

When done, remove the lid from the pot, then remove the pot from heat and let lentils stand for 15 minutes.

Meanwhile, switch on the oven, then set it to 350 degrees F and let it preheat.

Take a small bowl, place flaxseed in it, stir in water and let the mixture for 10 minutes until thickened.

Cook the vegetables and for this, take a medium skillet pan, place it over medium heat, add onion, garlic, celery, carrot, and bell pepper and then cook for 5 minutes.

Add all the spices, stir until well mixed, cook for 1 minute and then remove the pan from heat.

When lentils have cooled, use a fork to mash them until broken, add cooked vegetables, oats, flaxseed eggs, oat flour, salt, black pepper and stir well until combined.

Take a loaf pan, line it with parchment paper, and then spoon in prepared loaf mixture, pressing the filling into the pan.

Prepare the glaze and for this, take a small bowl, place all of its ingredients in it and stir until combined.

Spread the glaze over the top of the loaf, then bake for 45 minutes until cooked, and when done, let the loaf cool for 10 minutes.

Take out loaf from the pan, cut it into eight slices, and then serve.

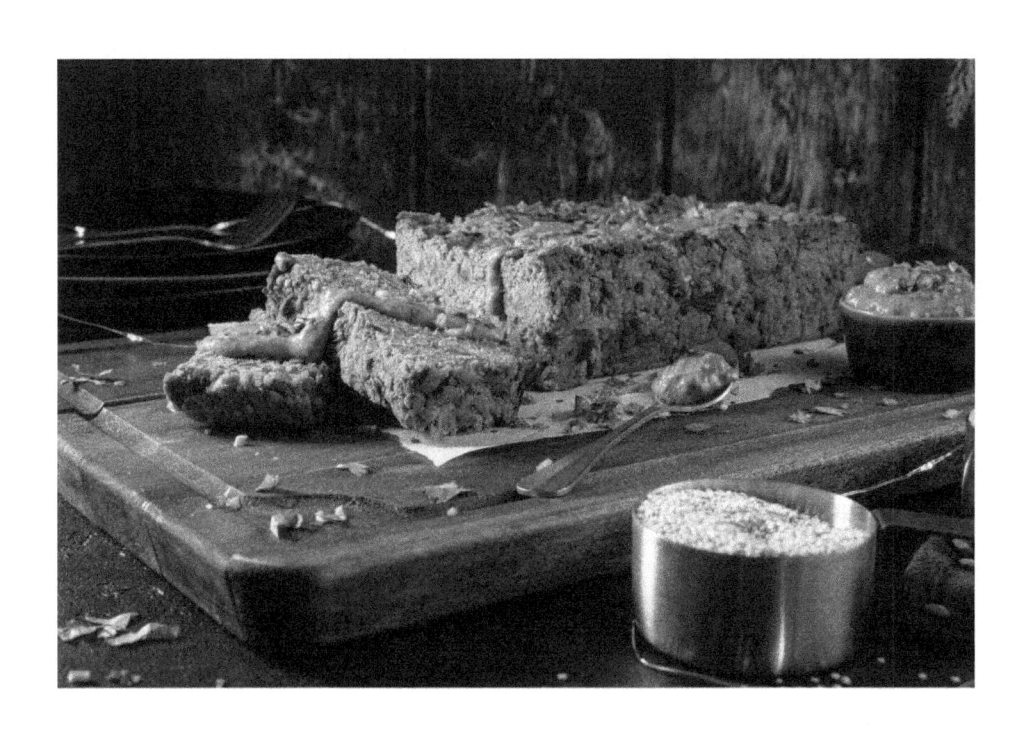

Mongolian Seitan

Serving: 6
Nutrition:
324 Cal; 8 g Fat; 1 g Saturated Fat; 33 g Carbohydrates; 3 g Fiber; 19 g Sugars; 29 g Protein;
Preparation time: 10 minutes
Cooking time: 20 minutes
Ingredients:
For the Sauce:
1 tablespoon minced garlic
1/2 teaspoon grated ginger
1/2 cup and 2 tablespoons coconut sugar
1/3 teaspoon red pepper flakes
1/3 teaspoon Chinese five-spice
2 teaspoons cornstarch
2 teaspoons olive oil
1/2 cup soy sauce
2 tablespoons cold water
For the Seitan:
1 pound seitan, 1-inch pieced
1 1/2 tablespoon olive oil
For Serving:
2 scallions, sliced
2 teaspoons toasted sesame seeds
Directions:
Prepare the sauce and for this, take a small saucepan, place it over medium heat, add oil and when hot, add ginger and garlic and cook for 30 seconds until fragrant.
Add red pepper flakes and the five-spice, continue cooking for 30 seconds, stir in sugar and soy sauce, then switch heat to medium-low level and simmer for 7 minutes until the sugar has dissolved and the sauce has slightly reduced.

Meanwhile, prepare the seitan and for this, take a large skillet pan, place it over medium-high heat, add oil and when hot, add seitan pieces and cook for 5 minutes until golden brown and edges have turned crispy.

Stir together cornstarch and water, add to the saucepan, stir until combined, and then cook for 3 minutes until the sauce has thickened slightly.

Switch heat to the low level, add seitan pieces, toss until well coated, and cook for 2 minutes until hot.

Sprinkle seitan with sesame seeds and scallions and then serve with cooked rice.

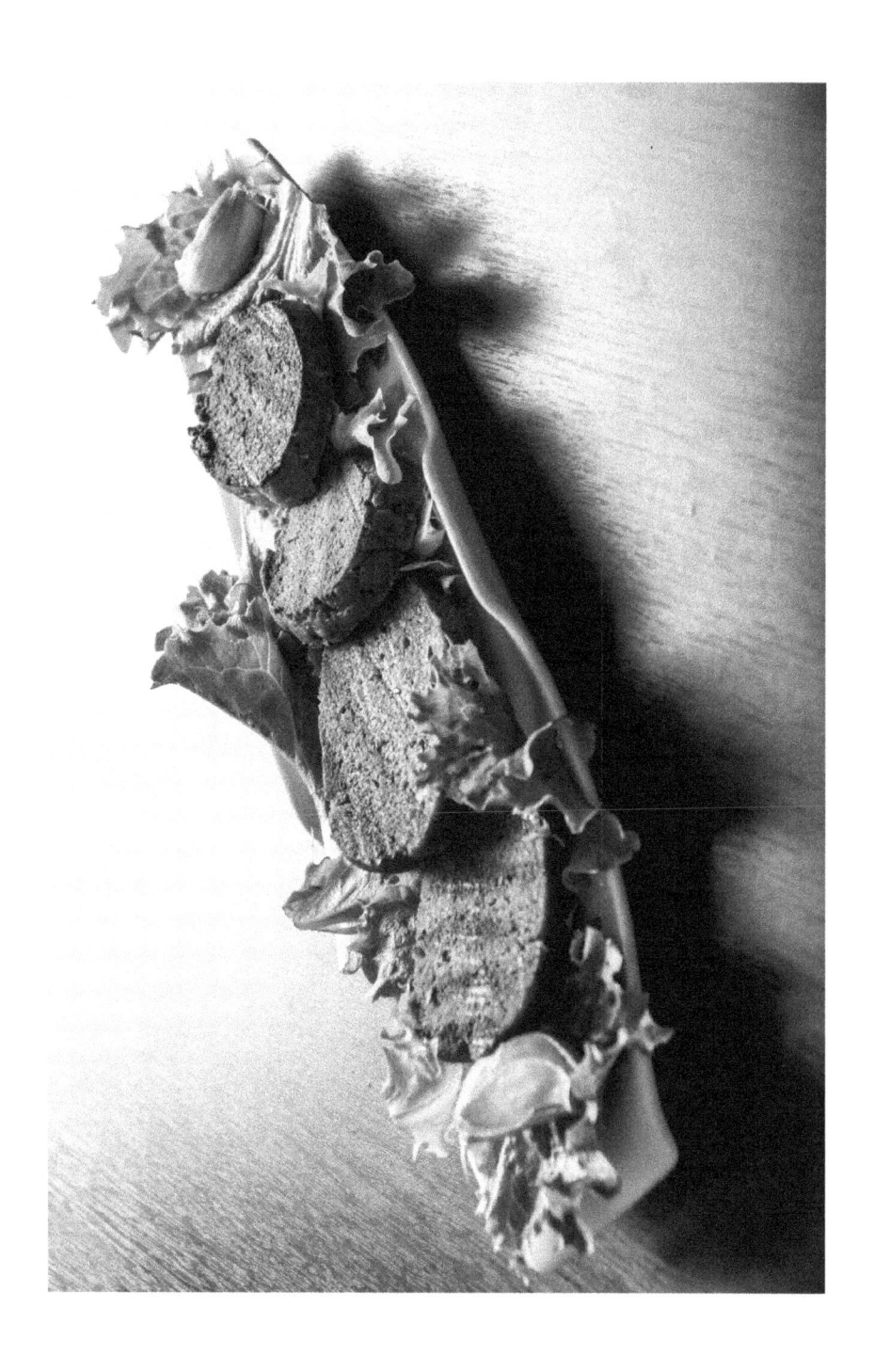

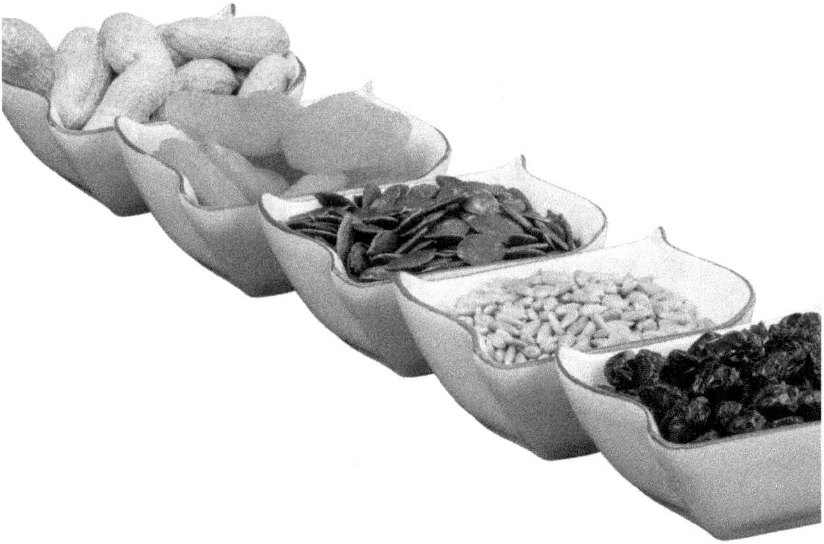

Snacks

Beans with Sesame Hummus

Preparation Time: 10 minutes
Servings: 6
Ingredients
4 Tbsp sesame oil
2 cloves garlic finely sliced
1 can (15 oz) cannellini beans, drained
4 Tbsp sesame paste
2 Tbsp lemon juice freshly squeezed
1/4 tsp red pepper flakes
2 Tbsp fresh basil finely chopped
2 Tbsp fresh parsley finely chopped
Sea salt to taste
Directions:
Place all ingredients in your food processor.
Process until all ingredients are combined well and smooth.
Transfer mixture into a bowl and refrigerate until servings.

Choco Walnuts Fat Bombs

Preparation Time: 15 minutes
Servings: 6
Ingredients
1/2 cup coconut butter
1/2 cup coconut oil softened
4 Tbs cocoa powder, unsweetened
4 Tbs brown sugar firmly packed
1/3 cup silken tofu mashed
1 cup walnuts, roughly chopped
Directions:
Add coconut butter and coconut oil into a microwave dish; melt it for 10-15 seconds.
Add in cocoa powder and whisk well.
Pour mixture into a blender with brown sugar and silken tofu cream; blend for 3-4 minutes.
Place silicone molds onto a sheet pan and fill halfway with chopped walnuts.
Pour the mixture over the walnuts and place it in the freezer for 6 hours.
Ready! Serve!
Nutrition:
Percent daily values based on the Reference Daily Intake (RDI) for a 2000 calorie diet.

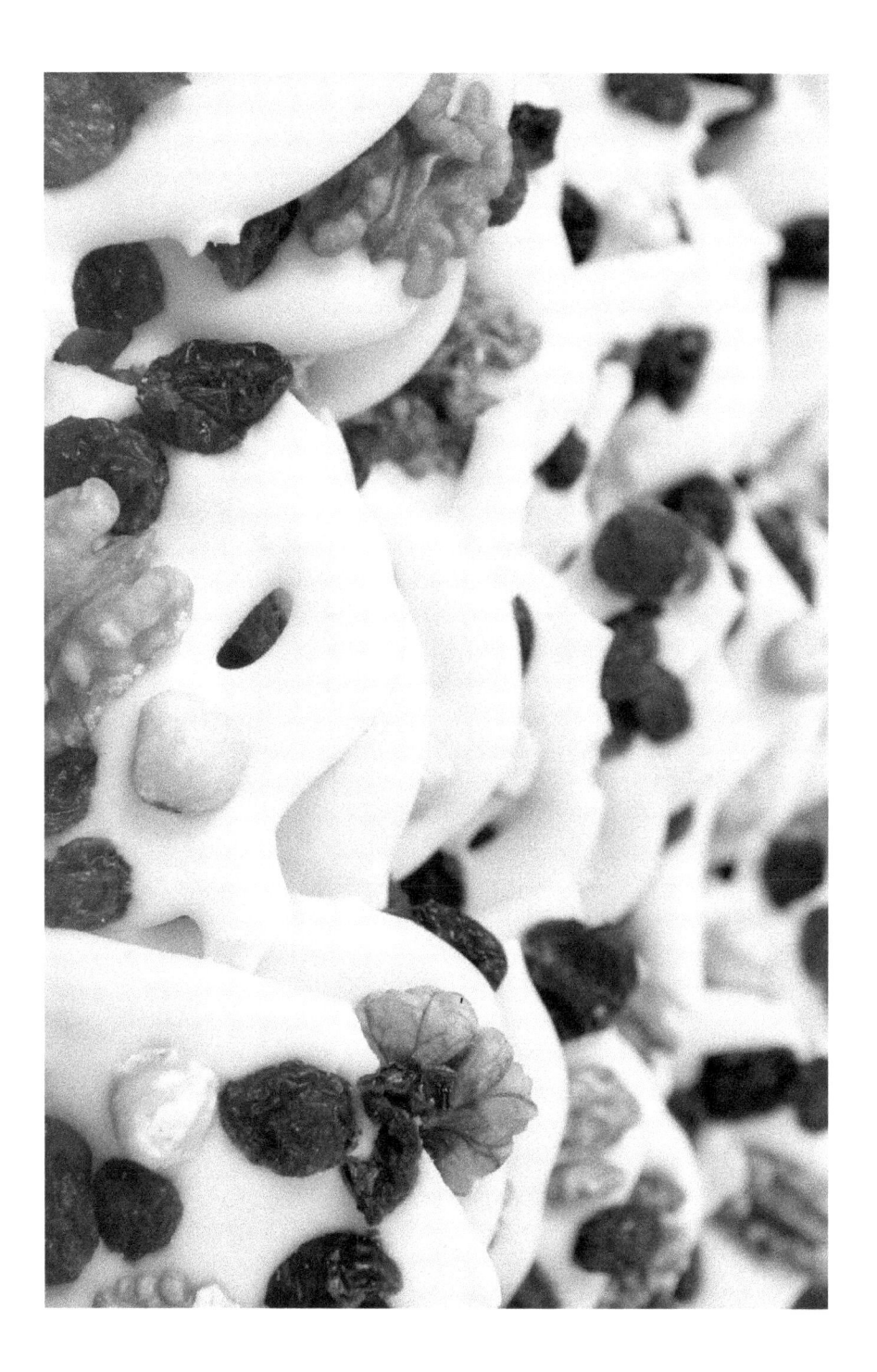

Crispy Honey Pecans (Slow Cooker)

Preparation Time: 2 hours and 15 minutes
Servings: 4
 Ingredients
16 oz pecan halves
4 Tbsp coconut butter melted
4 to 5 Tbsp honey strained
1/4 tsp ground ginger
1/4 tsp ground allspice
1 1/2 tsp ground cinnamon
Directions:
Add pecans and melted coconut butter into your 4-quart Slow Cooker.
Stir until combined well.
Add in honey and stir well.
In a bowl, combine spices and sprinkle over nuts; stir lightly.
Cook on LOW uncovered for about 2 to 3 hours or until nuts are crispy.
Serve cold.

Crunchy Fried Pickles

Preparation Time: 5 minutes
Servings: 6
Ingredients
1/2 cup Vegetable oil for frying
1 cup all-purpose flour
1 cup plain breadcrumbs
Pinch of salt and pepper
30 pickle chips (cucumber, dill)
Directions:
Heat oil in a large frying skillet over medium-high heat.
Stir the flour, breadcrumbs, and the salt and pepper in a shallow bowl.
Dredge the pickles in the flour/breadcrumbs mixture to coat completely.
Fry in batches until golden brown on all sides, 2 to 3 minutes in total.
Drain on paper towels and serve.

Granola bars with Maple Syrup

Preparation Time: 15 minutes
Servings: 12
Ingredients
3/4 cup dates chopped
2 Tbsp chia seeds soaked
3/4 cup rolled oats
4 Tbsp Chopped nuts such Macadamia, almond, Brazilian...etc,
2 Tbsp shredded coconut
2 Tbsp pumpkin seeds
2 Tbsp sesame seeds
2 Tbsp hemp seeds
1/2 cup maple syrup (or to taste)
1/4 cup peanut butter
Directions:
Add all ingredients (except maple syrup and peanut butter) into a food processor and pulse just until roughly combined.
Add maple syrup and peanut butter and process until all ingredients are combined well.
Place baking paper onto a medium baking dish and spread the mixture.
Cover with a plastic wrap and press down to make it flat.
Chill granola in the fridge for one hour.
Cut it into 12 bars and serve.
Keep stored in an airtight container for up to 1 week.
Also, you can wrap them individually in parchment paper, and keep in the freezer in a large Ziploc bag.

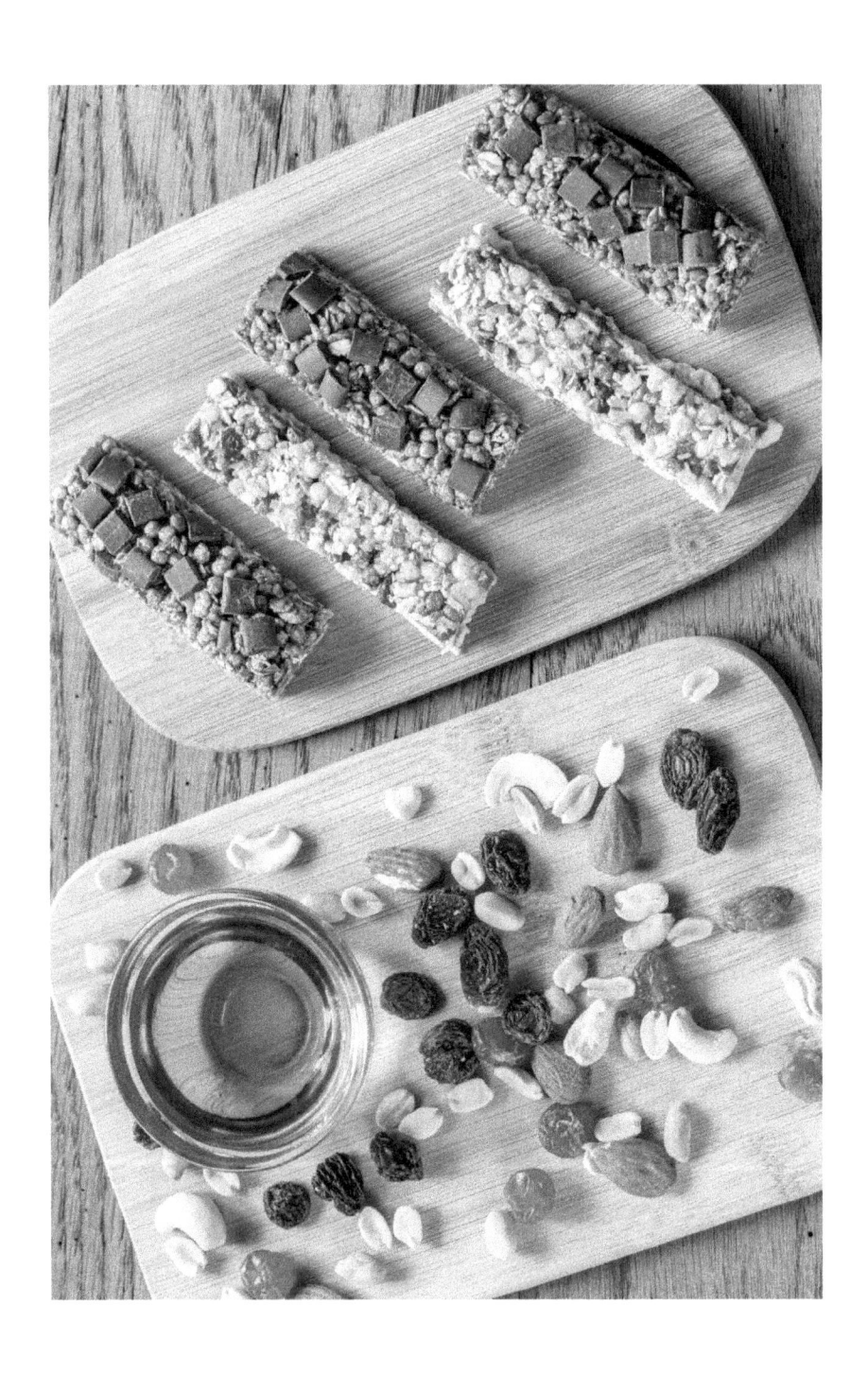

Green Soy Beans Hummus

Preparation Time: 15 minutes
Servings: 6
Ingredients
1 1/2 cups frozen green soybeans
4 cups of water
coarse salt to taste
1/4 cup sesame paste
1/2 tsp grated lemon peel
3 Tbsp fresh lemon juice
2 cloves of garlic crushed
1/2 tsp ground cumin
1/4 tsp ground coriander
4 Tbsp extra virgin olive oil
1 Tbsp fresh parsley leaves chopped
Serving options: sliced cucumber, celery, olives
Directions:
In a saucepan, bring to boil 4 cups of water with 2 to 3 pinch of coarse salt.
Add in frozen soybeans, and cook for 5 minutes or until tender.
Rinse and drain soybeans into a colander.
Add soybeans and all remaining ingredients into a food processor.
Pulse until smooth and creamy.
Taste and adjust salt to taste.
Serve with sliced cucumber, celery, olives, bread...etc.

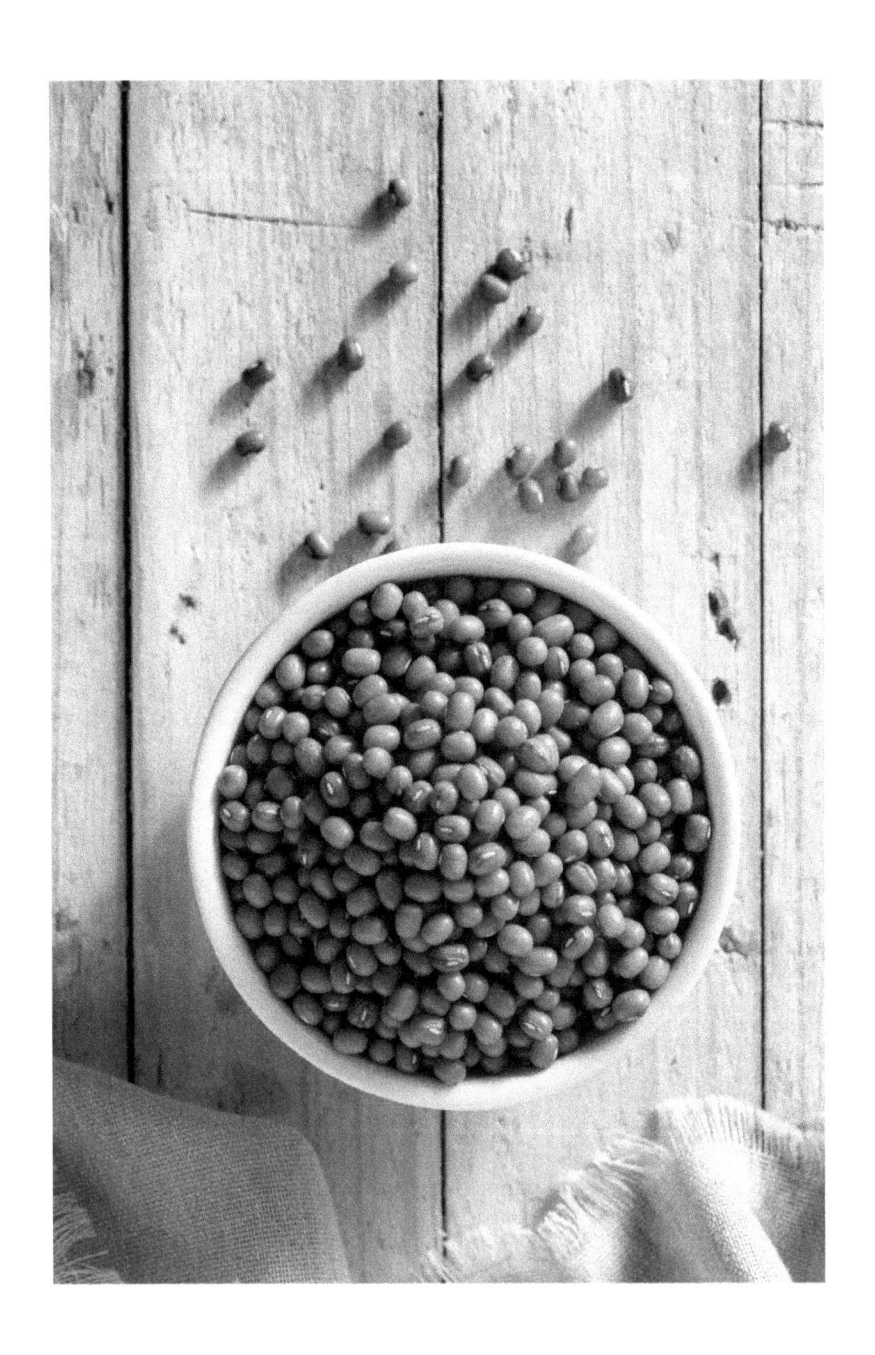

High Protein Avocado Guacamole

Preparation Time: 15 minutes
Servings: 4
Ingredients
1/2 cup of onion, finely chopped
1 chili pepper (peeled and finely chopped)
1 cup tomato, finely chopped
Cilantro leaves, fresh
2 avocados
2 Tbsp linseed oil
1/2 cup ground walnuts
1/2 lemon (or lime)
Salt
Directions:
Chop the onion, chili pepper, cilantro, and tomato; place in a large bowl.
Slice avocado, open vertically, and remove the pit.
Using the spoon take out the avocado flesh.
Mash the avocados with a fork and add into the bowl with onion mixture.
Add all remaining ingredients and stir well until ingredients combine well.
Taste and adjust salt and lemon/lime juice.
Keep refrigerated into covered glass bowl up to 5 days.

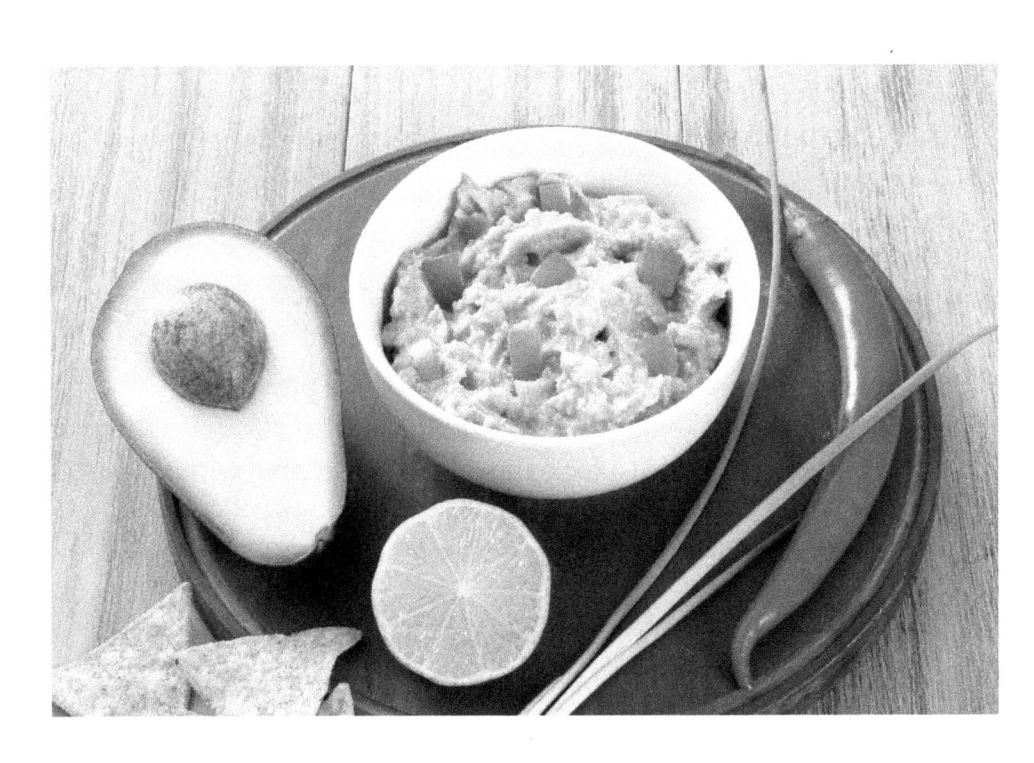

Homemade Energy Nut Bars

Preparation Time: 15 minutes
Servings: 4
Ingredients
1/2 cup peanuts
1 cup almonds
1/2 cup hazelnut, chopped
1 cup shredded coconut
1 cup almond butter
2 tsp sesame seeds toasted
1/2 cup coconut oil, freshly melted
2 Tbsp organic honey
1/4 tsp cinnamon
Directions:
Add all nuts into a food processor and pulse for 1-2 minutes.
Add in shredded coconut, almond butter, sesame seeds, melted coconut oil, cinnamon, and honey; process only for one minute.
Cover a square plate/tray with parchment paper and apply the nut mixture.
Spread mixture vigorously with a spatula.
Place in the freezer for 4 hours or overnight.
Remove from the freezer and cut into rectangular bars.
Ready! Enjoy!

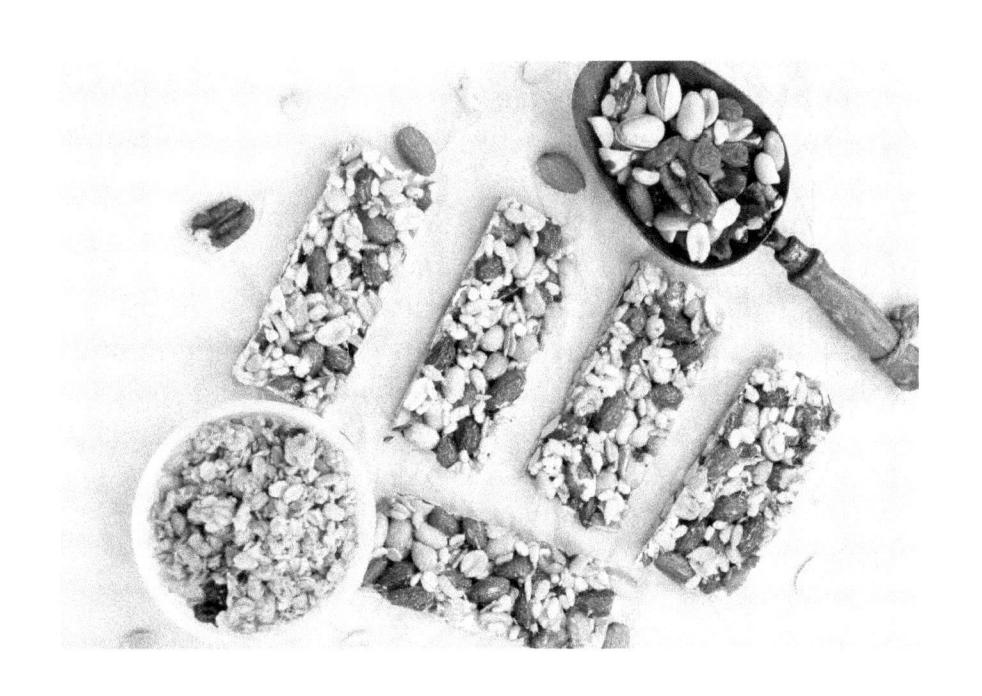

Honey Peanut Butter

Preparation Time: 10 minutes
Servings: 6
 Ingredients
1 cup peanut butter
3/4 cup honey extracted
1/2 cup ground peanuts
1 tsp ground cinnamon
Directions:
Add all ingredients into your fast-speed blender, and blend until smooth.
Keep refrigerated.

Mediterranean Marinated Olives

Preparation Time: 10 minutes
Servings: 2
Ingredients
24 large olives, black, green, Kalamata
1/2 cup extra-virgin olive oil
4 cloves garlic, thinly sliced
2 Tbsp fresh lemon juice
2 tsp coriander seeds, crushed
1/2 tsp crushed red pepper
1 tsp dried thyme
1 tsp dried rosemary, crushed
Salt and ground pepper to taste
Directions:
Place olives and all remaining ingredients in a large container or bag, and shake to combine well.
Cover and refrigerate to marinate overnight.
Serve.
Keep refrigerated.

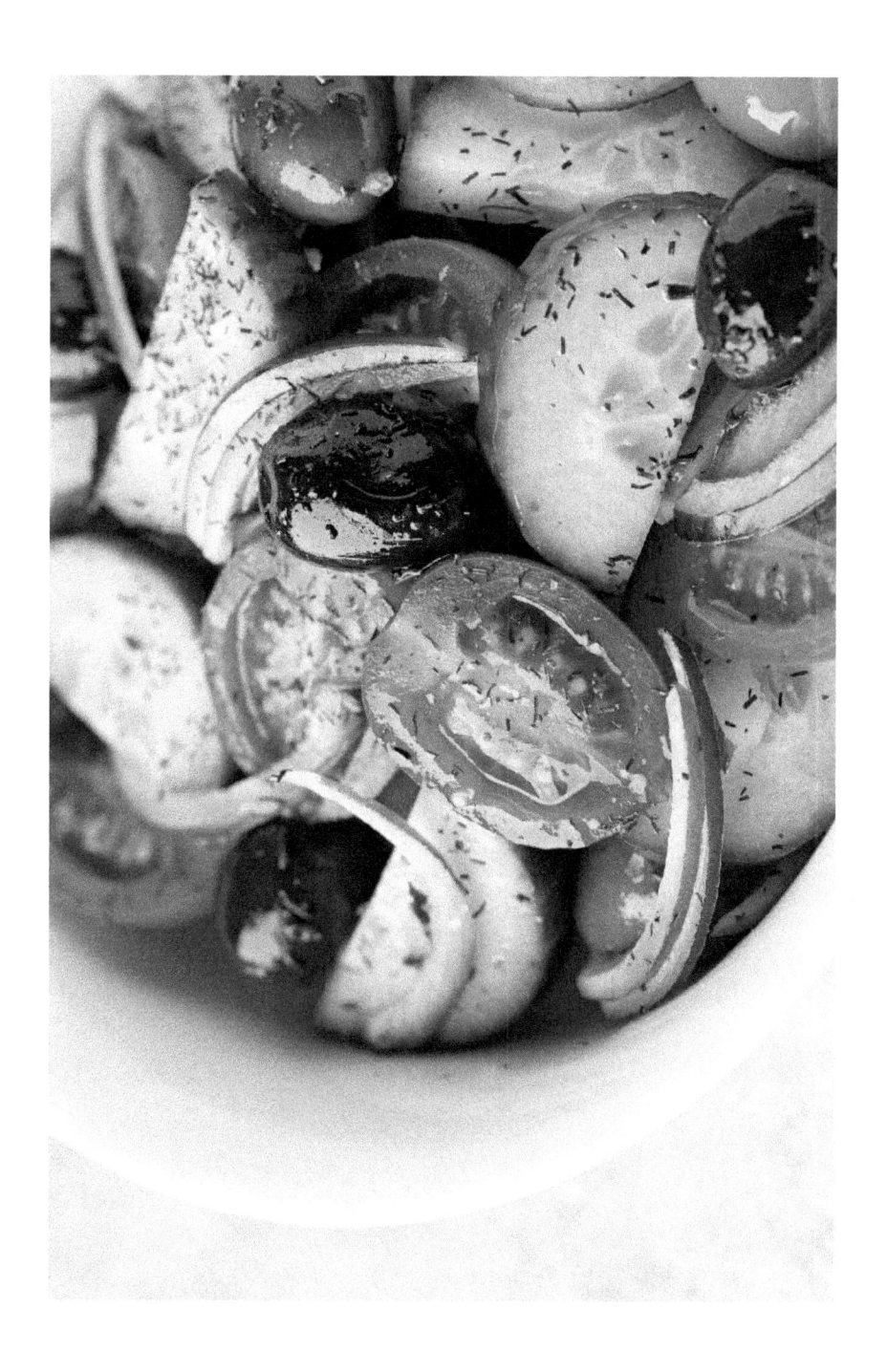

Pasta Recipes

Mushroom Cream Sauce Pasta

Servings: 4
Nutrition:
Calories: 998, Fat: 17 g, Carbohydrate: 179 g, Fiber: 14 g, Protein: 34 g
Ingredients:
4 tablespoons vegan margarine, divided
2 cloves garlic, peeled, minced
2 ½ cups soymilk or almond milk, unsweetened
Juice of a lemon
Freshly cracked pepper to taste
Salt to taste
24 ounces mushrooms of your choice, sliced
2 tablespoons flour
2 tablespoons chopped fresh parsley + extra to garnish
20 ounces cooked pasta (linguine or fettuccini)
Red pepper flakes to taste (optional)
Directions:
Place a heavy-bottomed pan over medium heat. Add 2 tablespoons margarine. When it melts, add mushrooms and garlic and sauté until soft. Transfer into a bowl and set aside.
Place the pan back over heat. Add remaining margarine. When it melts, add flour and constantly stir for about a minute.
Pour the milk you are using, whisking simultaneously. Keep stirring until thick.
Add the mushrooms, lemon juice, parsley, salt and pepper and heat for 3-4 minutes. Turn off the heat.
Divide pasta among 4 plates. Divide the sauce and spoon over the pasta.

Sprinkle parsley and red pepper flakes if using. Serve hot.
Tip: This sauce can also be served with cauliflower or tofu steaks or some vegan mock meat.

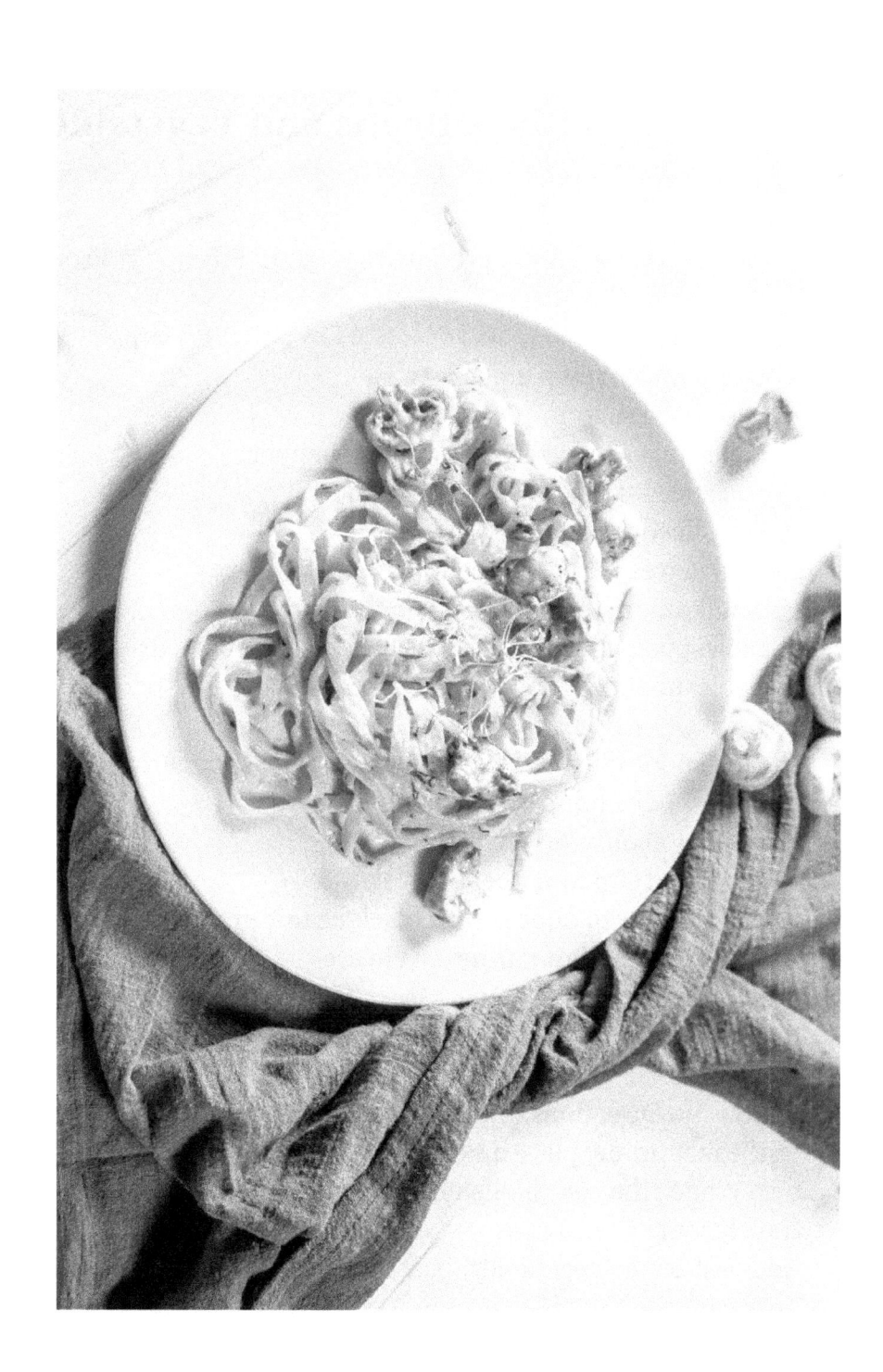

Penne with Black Beans and Vegetables

Servings: 3
Nutrition:
Calories: 315, Fat: 8 g, Carbohydrate: 50 g, Fiber: 7 g, Protein: 13 g
Ingredients:
5 ounces uncooked penne pasta
½ cup sliced carrots
¼ cup thinly sliced green or red bell pepper
¼ cup sliced fresh mushrooms
½ cup sliced zucchini
2 small cloves garlic, minced
½ small onion, thinly sliced
½ tablespoon chopped fresh basil, or 2 teaspoons dried basil
½ tablespoon chopped fresh oregano or 2 teaspoons dried oregano
½ tablespoon chopped fresh thyme, or 2 teaspoons dried thyme
½ tablespoon chopped fresh parsley
1 tablespoon olive oil, divided
1/3 chopped cup tomatoes
½ can (from a 15 ounces can) black beans, drained
3 tablespoons vegan Parmesan cheese
Salt to taste
Pepper to taste
Directions:
Follow the Directions: on the package and cook the pasta.
In the meantime, place a skillet over medium heat. Add half the oil. When the oil is heated, add onions and sauté until translucent.
Add rest of the vegetables, pasta, salt, dried herbs, and beans. Toss well.
Add tomatoes and toss well.
Drizzle the remaining oil and toss well.

Garnish with parsley and vegan cheese and serve.

Tofu Penne Pasta

Servings: 10
Nutrition:
Calories: 459, Fat: 13 g, Carbohydrate: 70 g, Fiber: NA g, Protein: 18 g
Ingredients:
For tofu:
4 square blocks, tofu, drained, pressed of excess moisture, crumbled into small pieces
2 teaspoons ground cumin
2 teaspoons garlic powder
3 tablespoons oil
1 cup soy sauce
½ teaspoon pepper
3 teaspoons chili powder
For pasta:
2 tablespoons canola oil
6 cloves garlic, pressed
8 teaspoons paprika or to taste
8 teaspoons garlic powder
8 teaspoons garlic powder
Cayenne pepper to taste
1 cup water
12 cups vegetable broth
10 cups dried penne pasta
2 large onions, diced
8 teaspoons dried oregano
8 teaspoons dried parsley
2 teaspoons salt or to taste
½ cup nutritional yeast
6 cups plant based milk of your choice, unsweetened
2 cans tomato sauce
3 cups frozen peas

For garnish: Optional
Vegan Parmesan cheese
Red pepper flakes
Chopped fresh parsley

Directions:

Add soy sauce, pepper, cumin, chili powder, oil, and garlic powder into a medium-size bowl. Whisk until well combined.

Add in the tofu. Let the tofu be well coated with the mixture.

Line a large baking sheet with parchment paper. Transfer the tofu onto the baking sheet. Spread it evenly.

Bake in a preheated oven at 400° F for 35-45 minutes or until firm. It will be meat-like in texture. Stir a couple of times while baking.

Remove from oven and set aside to cool.

Meanwhile, place a large Dutch oven over medium flame. Add oil. When the oil is heated, add onions and sauté until translucent.

Add garlic and cook until aromatic.

Add spices, herbs, salt, nutritional yeast, broth, milk, and tomato sauce and mix well.

When it begins to boil, add penne and cook until al dente. Stir often.

Turn off the heat. Add peas and tofu and stir. Let it sit for 10 minutes.

Garnish with the suggested garnishing's and serve.

Spinach Garlic Pasta

Servings: 4
Nutrition:
Calories: 188, Fat: 3.4 g, Carbohydrate: 33 g, Fiber: 3.1 g, Protein: 7.4 g
Ingredients:
½ package (from 16 ounces package) angel hair pasta
½ package (from 10 ounces package) frozen chopped spinach, thawed
2 large cloves garlic, minced
½ tablespoon olive oil
Salt to taste
Pepper to taste
Directions:
Follow the directions on the package and cook the pasta.
Place a skillet over medium heat. Add oil. When the oil is heated, add garlic and sauté for a few seconds until aromatic.
Add rest of the ingredients and toss well.
Serve hot.
Tip: You can use any pasta sauce if desired. I like my pasta simple, but my husband loves the pasta to be tossed in some pasta sauce.

Linguine with Guacamole

Servings: 4
Nutrition:
Calories: 450, Fat: 20 g, Carbohydrate: 49 g, Fiber: 13 g, Protein: 11 g
Ingredients:
8.1 ounces whole-wheat linguine
2 avocadoes, peeled, pitted, mashed
½ cup chopped fresh cilantro
2 small red chilies, deseeded, finely chopped
Juice of 2 limes
Zest of 2 limes, grated
4 large ripe tomatoes, finely chopped
2 red onions, finely chopped
Salt to taste
 Directions:
Follow the directions on the package and cook the pasta.
Meanwhile, add rest of the ingredients into a large bowl and stir.
Add pasta and toss well.
Serve warm or at room temperature. It also tastes great when chilled. Personally, I prefer chilled.

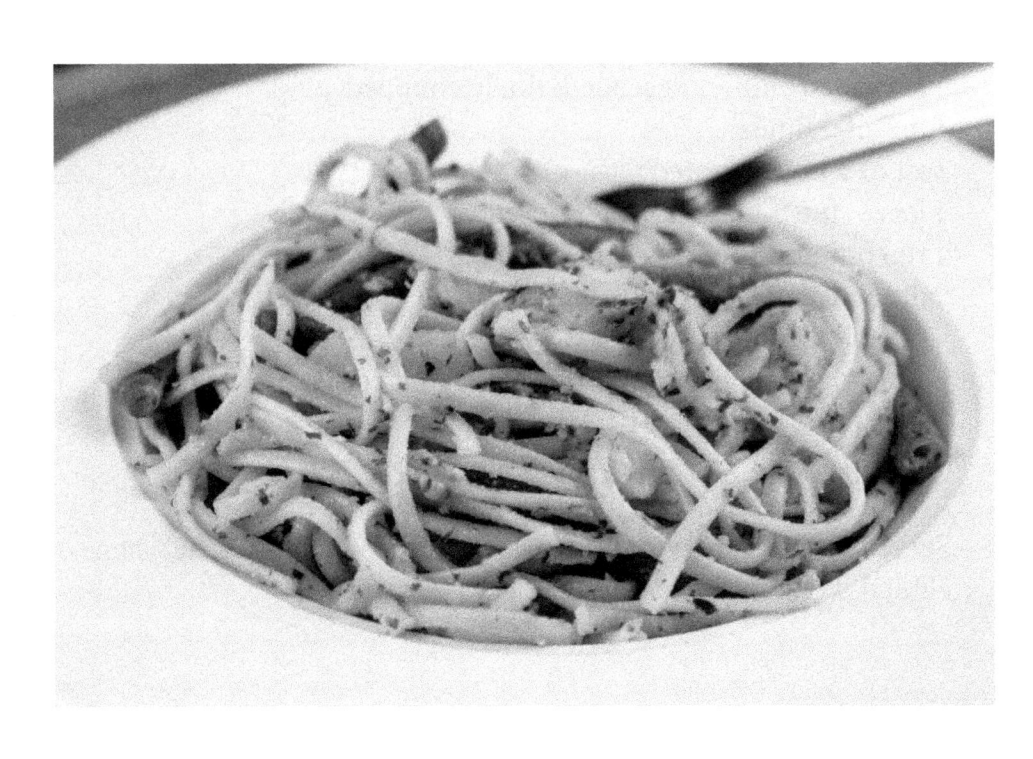

Dessert Recipes

Banana-Nut Bread Bars

Preparation time: 5 minutes
Cooking time: 30 minutes
Servings: 9 bars
Ingredients
Nonstick cooking spray (optional)
2 large ripe bananas
1 tablespoon maple syrup
½ Teaspoon vanilla extract
2 cups old-fashioned rolled oats
½ Teaspoons salt
¼ Cup chopped walnuts
Directions:
Preheat the oven to 350°f. Lightly coat a 9-by-9-inch baking pan with nonstick cooking spray (if using) or line with parchment paper for oil-free baking.
In a medium bowl, mash the bananas with a fork. Add the maple syrup and vanilla extract and mix well. Add the oats, salt, and walnuts, mixing well.
Transfer the batter to the baking pan and bake for 25 to 30 minutes, until the top is crispy. Cool completely before slicing into 9 bars. Transfer to an airtight storage container or a large plastic bag.
Nutrition (1 bar): calories: 73; fat: 1g; protein: 2g; carbohydrates: 15g; fiber: 2g; sugar: 5g; sodium: 129mg

Lemon Coconut Cilantro Rolls

Preparation time: 30 minutes • chill time: 30 minutes
Servings: 16 pieces
Ingredients
½ Cup fresh cilantro, chopped
1 cup sprouts (clover, alfalfa)
1 garlic clove, pressed
2 tablespoons ground brazil nuts or almonds
2 tablespoons flaked coconut
1 tablespoon coconut oil
Pinch cayenne pepper
Pinch sea salt
Pinch freshly ground black pepper
Zest and juice of 1 lemon
2 tablespoons ground flaxseed
1 to 2 tablespoons water
2 whole-wheat wraps, or corn wraps
Directions:
Put everything but the wraps in a food processor and pulse to combine. Or combine the Ingredients in a large bowl. Add the water, if needed, to help the mix come together.
Spread the mixture out over each wrap, roll it up, and place it in the fridge for 30 minutes to set.
Remove the rolls from the fridge and slice each into 8 pieces to serve as appetizers or sides with a soup or stew.
Get the best flavor by buying whole raw brazil nuts or almonds, toasting them lightly in a dry skillet or toaster oven, and then grinding them in a coffee grinder.
Nutrition (1 piece) calories: 66; total fat: 4g; carbs: 6g; fiber: 1g; protein: 2g

Tamari Almonds

Preparation time:5minutes
Cooking time:15minutes
Servings: 8
Ingredients
1 pound raw almonds
3 tablespoons tamari or soy sauce
2 tablespoons extra-virgin olive oil
1 tablespoon Nutritional yeast
1 to 2 teaspoons chili powder, to taste
Directions:
Preheat the oven to 400°f.
Line a baking sheet with parchment paper.
In a medium bowl, combine the almonds, tamari, and olive oil until well coated.
Spread the almonds on the prepared baking sheet and roast for 10 to 15 minutes, until browned.
Cool for 10 minutes, then season with the Nutritional yeast and chili powder.
Transfer to a glass jar and close tightly with a lid.
Nutrition: calories: 364; fat: 32g; protein: 13g; carbohydrates: 13g; fiber: 7g; sugar: 3g; sodium: 381mg

Tempeh Taco Bites

Preparation time: 5 minutes
Cooking time: 45 minutes
Servings: 3 dozen
Ingredients
8 ounces tempeh
3 tablespoons soy sauce
2 teaspoons ground cumin
1 teaspoon chili powder
1 teaspoon dried oregano
1 tablespoon olive oil
1/2 cup finely minced onion
2 garlic cloves, minced
Salt and freshly ground black pepper
2 tablespoons tomato paste
1 chipotle chile in adobo, finely minced
1/4 cup hot water or vegetable broth, homemade or store-bought, plus more if needed
36 phyllo pastry cups, thawed
1/2 cup basic guacamole, homemade or store-bought
18 ripe cherry tomatoes, halved
Directions
In a medium saucepan of simmering water, cook the tempeh for 30 minutes. Drain well, then finely mince and place it in a bowl. Add the soy sauce, cumin, chili powder, and oregano. Mix well and set aside.
In a medium skillet, heat the oil over medium heat. Add the onion, cover, and cook for 5 minutes. Stir in the garlic, then add the tempeh mixture and cook, stirring, for 2 to 3 minutes. Season with salt and pepper to taste. Set aside.

In a small bowl, combine the tomato paste, chipotle, and the hot water or broth. Return tempeh mixture to heat and in stir tomato-chile mixture and cook for 10 to 15 minutes, stirring occasionally, until the liquid is absorbed.

The mixture should be fairly dry, but if it begins to stick to the pan, add a little more hot water, 1 tablespoon at a time. Taste, adjusting seasonings if necessary. Remove from the heat.

To assemble, fill the phyllo cups to the top with the tempeh filling, using about 2 teaspoons of filling in each. Top with a dollop of guacamole and a cherry tomato half and serve.

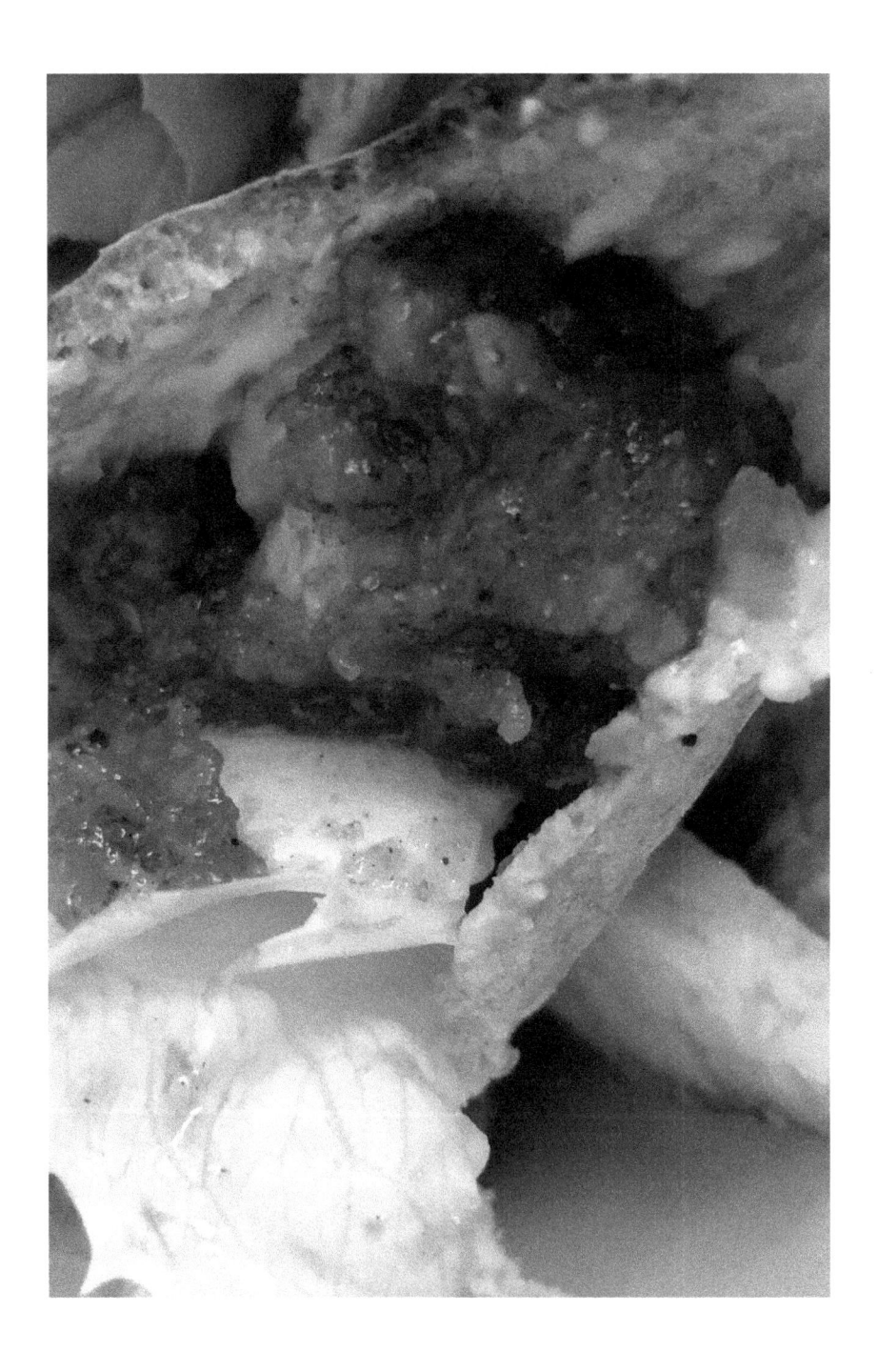

Stuffed Cherry Tomatoes

Preparation time:15minutes
Cooking time:0minutes
Servings: 6
Ingredients
2 pints cherry tomatoes, tops removed and centers scooped out
2 avocados, mashed
Juice of 1 lemon
½ Red bell pepper, minced
4 green onions (white and green parts), finely minced
1 tablespoon minced fresh tarragon
Pinch of sea salt
Directions:
Place the cherry tomatoes open-side up on a platter.
In a small bowl, combine the avocado, lemon juice, bell pepper, scallions, tarragon, and salt.
Stir until well combined. Scoop into the cherry tomatoes and serve immediately.

Spicy Black Bean Dip

Preparation time: 10 minutes
Cooking time: 0 minutes
Servings: 2 cups
Ingredients
1 (14-ounce) can black beans, drained and rinsed, or 1½ cups cooked
Zest and juice of 1 lime
1 tablespoon tamari, or soy sauce
¼ Cup water
¼ Cup fresh cilantro, chopped
1 teaspoon ground cumin
Pinch cayenne pepper
Directions:
Put the beans in a food processor (best choice) or blender, along with the lime zest and juice, tamari, and about ¼ cup of water. Blend until smooth, then blend in the cilantro, cumin, and cayenne.
If you don't have a blender or prefer a different consistency, simply transfer it to a bowl once the beans have been puréed and stir in the spices, instead of forcing the blender.
Nutrition (1 cup) calories: 190; total fat: 1g; carbs: 35g; fiber: 12g; protein: 13g

Cheezy Cashew–Roasted Red Pepper Toasts

Preparation time: 15 minutes
Cooking time: 0 minutes
Servings: 16 to 24 toasts
Ingredients
2 jarred roasted red peppers
1 cup unsalted cashews
1/4 cup water
1 tablespoon soy sauce
2 tablespoons chopped green onions
1/4 cup Nutritional yeast
2 tablespoons balsamic vinegar
2 tablespoons olive oil
Directions
Use canapé or cookie cutters to cut the bread into desired shapes about 2 inches wide. If you don't have a cutter, use a knife to cut the bread into squares, triangles, or rectangles. You should get 2 to 4 pieces out of each slice of bread. Toast the bread and set aside to cool.
Coarsely chop 1 red pepper and set aside. Cut the remaining pepper into thin strips or decorative shapes and set aside for garnish.
In a blender or food processor, grind the cashews to a fine powder. Add the water and soy sauce and process until smooth. Add the chopped red pepper and puree. Add the green onions, Nutritional yeast, vinegar, and oil and process until smooth and well blended.
Spread a spoonful of the pepper mixture onto each of the toasted bread pieces and top decoratively with the reserved pepper strips. Arrange on a platter or tray and serve.

Baked Potato Chips

Preparation time:10minutes
Cooking time:30minutes
Servings: 4
Ingredients
1 large russet potato
1 teaspoon paprika
½ Teaspoon garlic salt
¼ Teaspoon vegan sugar
¼ Teaspoon onion powder
¼ Teaspoon chipotle powder or chili powder
⅛ Teaspoon salt
⅛ Teaspoon ground mustard
⅛ Teaspoon ground cayenne pepper
1 teaspoon canola oil
⅛ Teaspoon liquid smoke
Directions:
Wash and peel the potato. Cut into thin, 1/10-inch slices (a mandoline slicer or the slicer blade in a food processor is helpful for consistently sized slices).
Fill a large bowl with enough very cold water to cover the potato. Transfer the potato slices to the bowl and soak for 20 minutes.
Preheat the oven to 400°f. Line a baking sheet with parchment paper.
In a small bowl, combine the paprika, garlic salt, sugar, onion powder, chipotle powder, salt, mustard, and cayenne.
Drain and rinse the potato slices and pat dry with a paper towel. Transfer to a large bowl.
Add the canola oil, liquid smoke, and spice mixture to the bowl. Toss to coat.
Transfer the potatoes to the prepared baking sheet.

Bake for 15 minutes. Flip the chips over and bake for 15 minutes longer, until browned. Transfer the chips to 4 storage containers or large glass jars.
Let cool before closing the lids tightly.
Nutrition: calories: 89; fat: 1g; protein: 2g; carbohydrates: 18g; fiber: 2g; sugar: 1g; sodium: 65mg

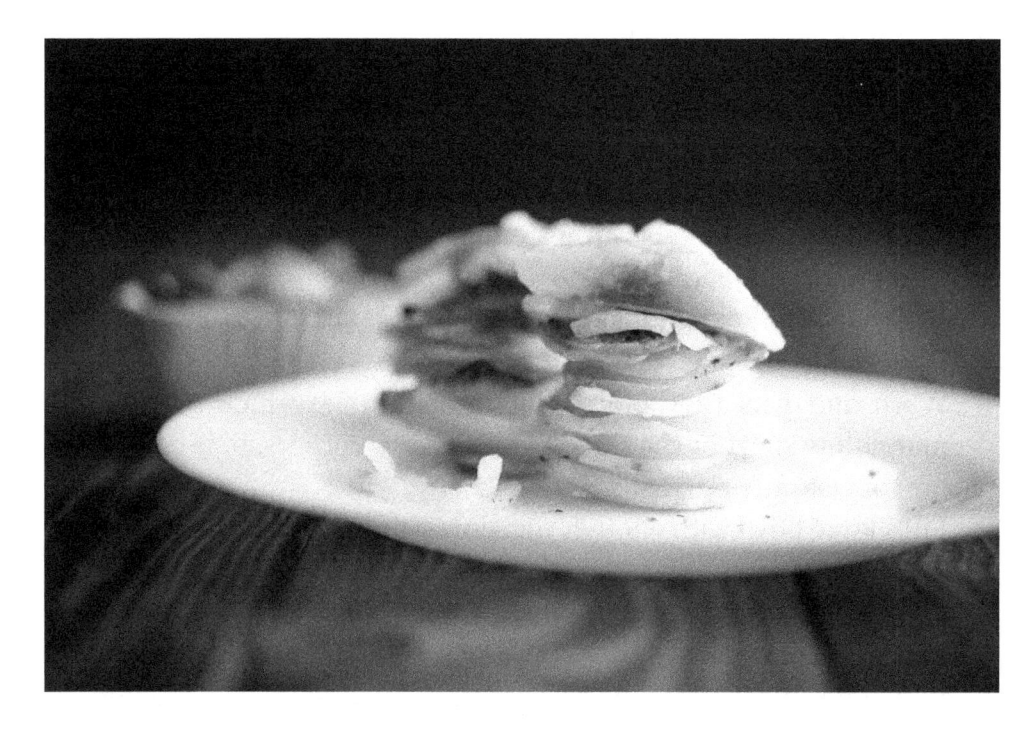

Mushrooms Stuffed With Spinach And Walnuts

Preparation time: 10 minutes
Cooking time: 6 minutes
Servings: 4 to 6 servings
Ingredients
2 tablespoons olive oil
8 ounces white mushroom, lightly rinsed, patted dry, and stems reserved
1 garlic clove, minced
1 cup cooked spinach
1 cup finely chopped walnuts
1/2 cup unseasoned dry bread crumbs
Salt and freshly ground black pepper
Directions
Preheat the oven to 400°f. Lightly oil a large baking pan and set aside. In a large skillet, heat the oil over medium heat. Add the mushroom caps and cook for 2 minutes to soften slightly. Remove from the skillet and set aside.
Chop the mushroom stems and add to the same skillet. Add the garlic and cook over medium heat until softened, about 2 minutes. Stir in the spinach, walnuts, bread crumbs, and salt and pepper to taste. Cook for 2 minutes, stirring well to combine.
Fill the reserved mushroom caps with the stuffing mixture and arrange in the baking pan. Bake until the mushrooms are tender and the filling is hot, about 10 minutes. Serve hot.

Salsa Fresca

Preparation time: 15 minutes
Cooking time: 0 minutes
Servings: 4

Ingredients

3 large heirloom tomatoes or other fresh tomatoes, chopped
½ Red onion, finely chopped
½ Bunch cilantro, chopped
2 garlic cloves, minced
1 jalapeño, minced
Juice of 1 lime, or 1 tablespoon prepared lime juice
¼ Cup olive oil
Sea salt
Whole-grain tortilla chips, for serving

Directions:

In a small bowl, combine the tomatoes, onion, cilantro, garlic, jalapeño, lime juice, and olive oil and mix well. Allow to sit at room temperature for 15 minutes. Season with salt.

Serve with tortilla chips.

The salsa can be stored in an airtight container in the refrigerator for up to 1 week.

Guacamole

Preparation time:10minutes
Cooking time:0minutes
Servings: 2
Ingredients
2 ripe avocados
2 garlic cloves, pressed
Zest and juice of 1 lime
1 teaspoon ground cumin
Pinch sea salt
Pinch freshly ground black pepper
Pinch cayenne pepper (optional)
Directions:
Mash the avocados in a large bowl. Add the rest of the Ingredients and stir to combine.
Try adding diced tomatoes (cherry are divine), chopped scallions or chives, chopped fresh cilantro or basil, lemon rather than lime, paprika, or whatever you think would taste good!
Nutrition (1 cup) calories: 258; total fat: 22g; carbs: 18g; fiber: 11g; protein: 4g

Asian Lettuce Rolls

Preparation time:15minutes
Cooking time:5minutes
Servings: 4
Ingredients
2 ounces rice noodles
2 tablespoons chopped thai basil
2 tablespoons chopped cilantro
1 garlic clove, minced
1 tablespoon minced fresh ginger
Juice of ½ lime, or 2 teaspoons prepared lime juice
2 tablespoons soy sauce
1 cucumber, julienned
2 carrots, peeled and julienned
8 leaves butter lettuce
Directions:
Cook the rice noodles according to package Directions.
In a small bowl, whisk together the basil, cilantro, garlic, ginger, lime juice, and soy sauce. Toss with the cooked noodles, cucumber, and carrots.
Divide the mixture evenly among lettuce leaves and roll.
Secure with a toothpick and serve immediately.

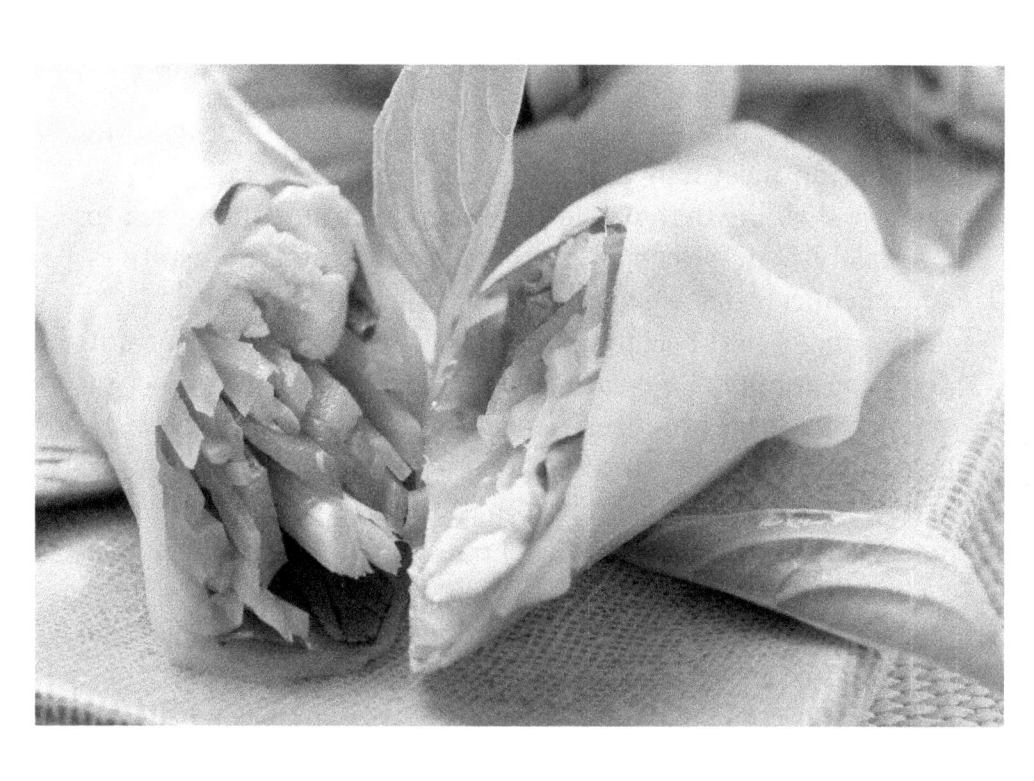

Conclusion

As you become more aware of the nutritional benefits of your food, you will also notice the quality and not the quantity consumed daily matters. We can learn to make more eco-conscious decisions of where our food comes from, how its production affects our environment and consumption, when and where to buy local produce, reduce our waste and learn how we can localize our own production and harvest of crops, right in our homes.

In the long run, we can also choose to save money from purchasing meat and dairy products which generally have a shorter shelf life than plants-based products and often need to be replenished. We can be mindful of the harmful preservatives and chemicals that we have been putting into our bodies.

As we move into becoming more socially responsible for our food consumption, we can have a larger purchasing power of supporting local producers that reduce their ecological waste and thumbprint. We can also choose to pay to support fair trade workers along the production line of our favourite imported goods, choose produce only in the season to reduce our intake of genetically-modified products and pesticides, and purchase just enough to be consumed according to the natural shelf life and cycle of our products.

Furthermore, by starting to consume more plants, you will also start to realize the natural benefits of its derivatives serving anti-bacterial and anti-septic properties in household cleaners, storage units, skincare products, and more!

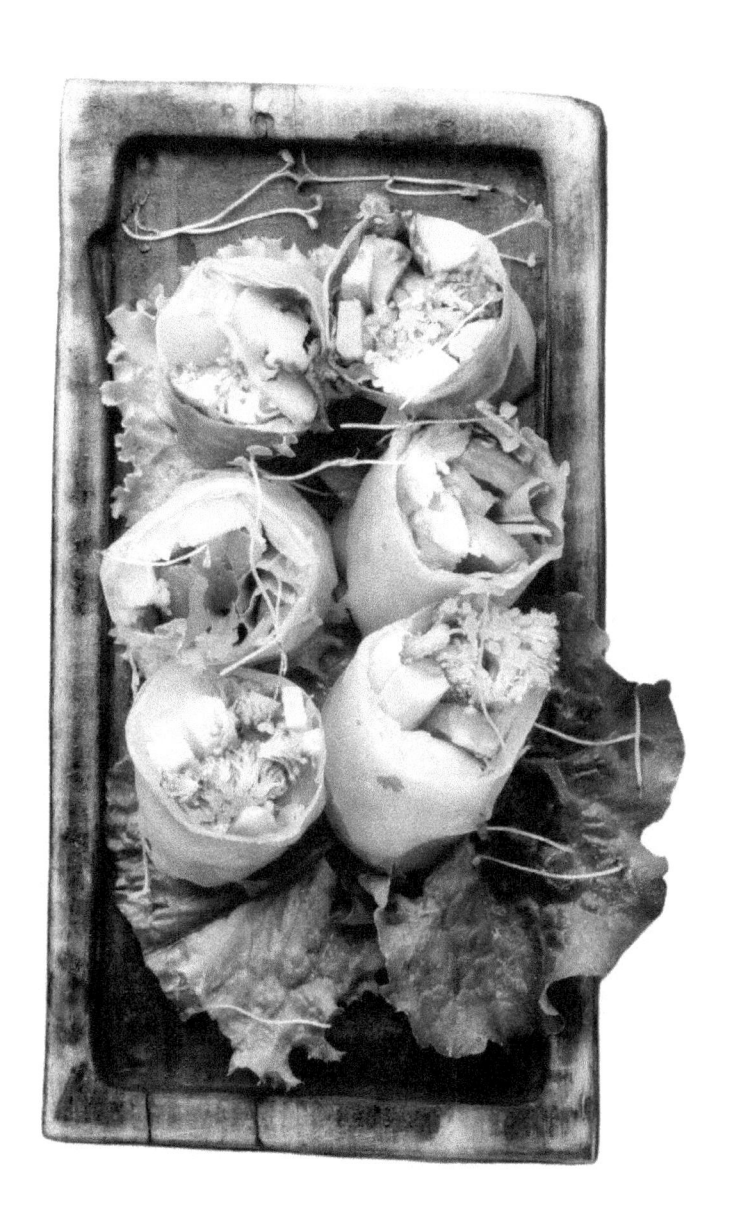

Lightning Source UK Ltd.
Milton Keynes UK
UKHW051008310521
384576UK00013B/305